# THE
# AUTOIMMUNE
# PROTOCOL
## MADE SIMPLE
### COOKBOOK

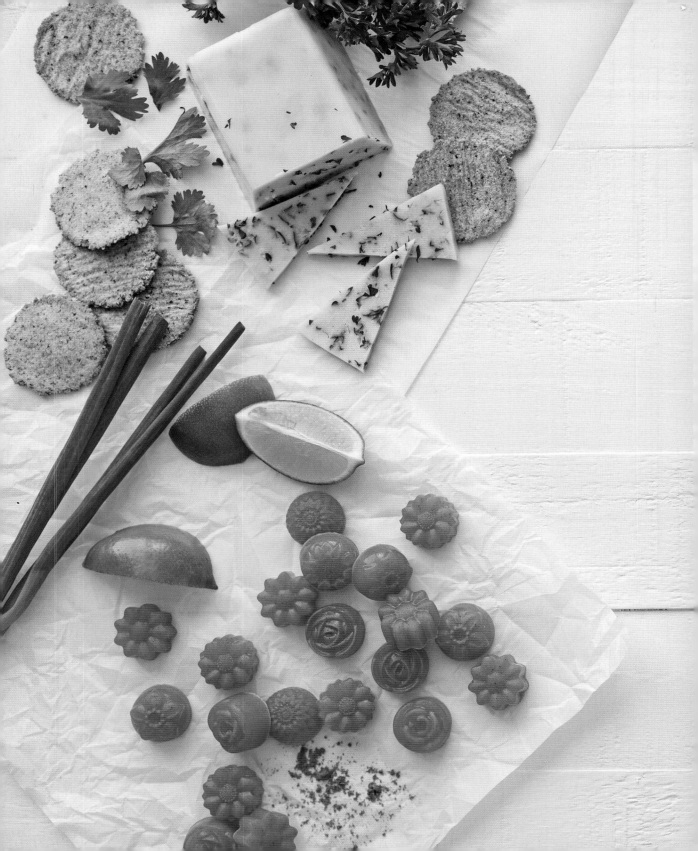

# THE
# AUTOIMMUNE
# PROTOCOL
# MADE SIMPLE

## COOKBOOK

### Start Healing Your Body *and* Reversing Chronic Illness Today *with* 100 Delicious Recipes

SOPHIE VAN TIGGELEN

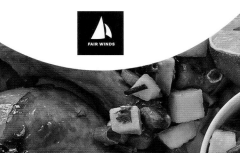

FAIR WINDS

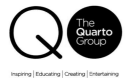

Inspiring | Educating | Creating | Entertaining

Brimming with creative inspiration, how-to projects, and useful information to enrich your everyday life, quarto.com is a favorite destination for those pursuing their interests and passions.

© 2018 Quarto Publishing Group USA Inc.

Text © 2018 Sophie Van Tiggelen

Photography © 2018 Lisa Patchem Photography

First Published in 2018 by Fair Winds Press, an imprint of The Quarto Group,

100 Cummings Center, Suite 265-D, Beverly, MA 01915, USA.

T (978) 282-9590 F (978) 283-2742 Quarto.com

Fair Winds Press titles are also available at discount for retail, wholesale, promotional, and bulk purchase. For details, contact the Special Sales Manager by email at specialsales@quarto.com or by mail at The Quarto Group, Attn: Special Sales Manager, 100 Cummings Center, Suite 265-D, Beverly, MA 01915, USA.

23          10

ISBN: 978-1-59233-817-7

Digital edition published in 2018

Library of Congress Cataloging-in-Publication Data

Tiggelen, Sophie Van, author.

The autoimmune protocol made simple cookbook : start healing your body

  and reversing chronic illness today with 100 delicious recipes / Sophie

  Van Tiggelen.

ISBN 9781592338177 (paperback)

1.  Autoimmune diseases--Treatment. 2. Autoimmune diseases--Diet

  therapy. 3. Autoimmune diseases--Diet therapy--Recipes.

RC600 .T54 2018

641.5/631--dc23

2017059558

Design: Stacy Wakefield-Forte

Cover Images: Lisa Patchem Photography

Page Layout: Stacy Wakefield-Forte

Photography: Lisa Patchem Photography

Printed in China

The information in this book is for educational purposes only. It is not intended to replace the advice of a physician or medical practitioner. Please see your health-care provider before beginning any new health program.

*dedication*

THIS BOOK IS DEDICATED TO ALL AUTOIMMUNE WARRIORS.
"THE NATURAL HEALING FORCE WITHIN EACH OF US IS THE GREATEST
FORCE IN GETTING WELL."—HIPPOCRATES

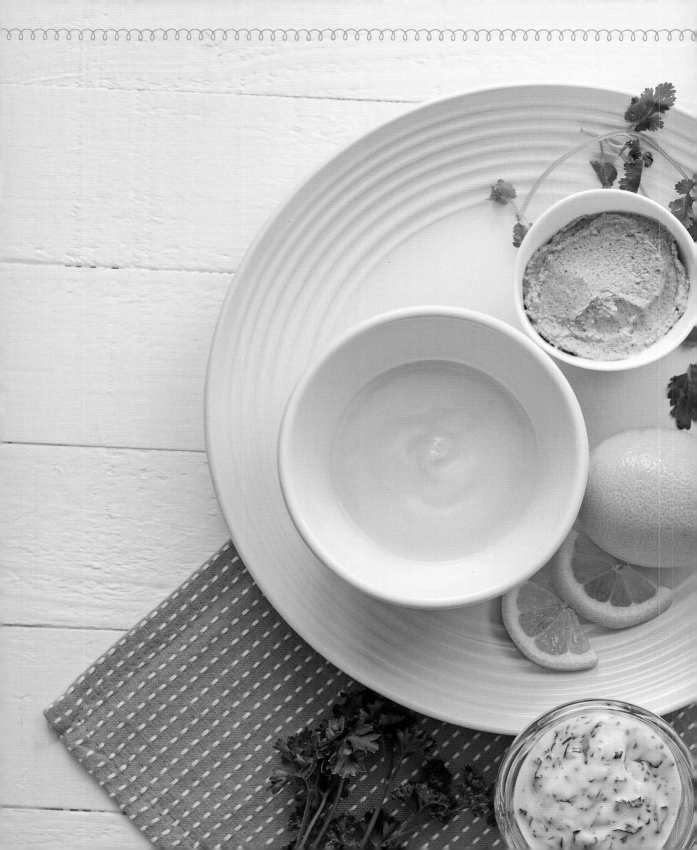

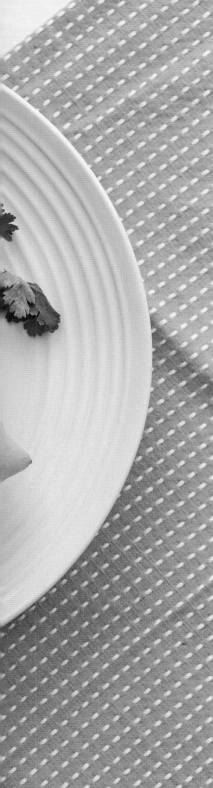

**AUTOIMMUNE DISEASE** is an epidemic in our society, affecting an estimated 50 million Americans. There are more than 100 confirmed autoimmune diseases—some of the most common being Grave's disease, Hashimoto's thyroiditis, lupus, rheumatoid arthritis, multiple sclerosis, Sjögren's syndrome, alopecia, psoriasis, ulcerative colitis, Crohn's disease, and type 1 diabetes. All autoimmune diseases have the same root cause: Our immune system, which is supposed to protect us from pathogens, turns against us and attacks our own proteins, cells, and tissues. The specific tissues attacked determine which autoimmune disease you have. These conditions are chronic and lifelong and many come with debilitating symptoms that can rob us of our quality of life.

Genetics account for about one third of our risk for autoimmune disease; the rest comes from environmental exposures—like infection, toxins, and pollutants—diet, and lifestyle. The good news: Immune function is very sensitive to diet and lifestyle choices. That means, with the right diet and lifestyle choices, we can modulate the immune system to increase immunoregulatory processes in the body with the net effect of reducing the inflammation and targeted immune attacks on our tissues that drive autoimmune disease.

What are the right diet and lifestyle choices to mitigate autoimmune disease? The answer is the recommendations of the Autoimmune Protocol, or AIP.

The Autoimmune Protocol is a template for selecting foods and prioritizing life-style factors to maximize the therapeutic potential of our day-to-day choices. Each facet is supported by scientific evidence, making the AIP a valuable complementary approach to chronic disease management. In a 2017 clinical trial in patients with Inflammatory Bowel Disease, 73 percent of participants were in full clinical remission after following the protocol for only six weeks, and they experienced continued improvement over the entire course of the study.

*The Autoimmune Protocol Made Simple Cookbook*

The Autoimmune Protocol focuses on providing the body with the nutritional resources required for immune regulation and tissue healing while removing inflammatory stimuli from both diet and lifestyle. The AIP diet provides balanced and complete nutrition while avoiding processed and refined foods and empty calories. The immune system requires a vast array of nutrients to function properly, which is why the AIP diet homes in on the most nutrient-dense whole foods available in the food supply—including seafood, organ meat, and at least eight servings of vegetables per day. However, the food on our plate isn't the only input to health. The AIP lifestyle encourages sufficient sleep, stress management, and activity, as these are also important immune modulators, both directly and indirectly, for example by affecting gut health. Together, the diet and lifestyle guidelines of the Autoimmune Protocol support a healthy gut, including a diverse gut microbiome, hormone regulation, and immune regulation, all essential for lifelong health and wellness.

Whether you are just beginning your health journey or are looking for inspiration in the kitchen to propel your healing forward, *The Autoimmune Protocol Made Simple Cookbook* is a fantastic resource! With 100 delicious AIP recipes that are both creative and easy-to-make, Sophie Van Tiggelen has ensured that you won't feel like you're eating a restricted diet. And thanks to diet guidelines, shopping lists, and an excellent summary of the AIP with a focus on actionable information, you can jump right into the Autoimmune Protocol with this book.

Health and wellness after an autoimmune diagnosis requires attention to the foods we eat and how we structure our lives, but it doesn't need to be hard or leave us feeling deprived. And with this book at your fingertips, you'll love getting into the kitchen, cooking nourishing AIP meals, and savoring every bite!

—Sarah Ballantyne, Ph.D.,
*New York Times* bestselling author of
*The Paleo Approach* and *Paleo Principles*

# CHAPTER ONE

# GETTING STARTED ON THE AIP DIET

**THE FOOD WE EAT** fuels our bodies and affects every function from our metabolism to our immunity. If we consume food that is less than healthy, over time, our bodies will begin to feel the effects of it and not function optimally. On the other hand, if we fuel ourselves with the best, most nutrient-dense food we can afford, our bodies will feel the difference almost immediately. The idea of using nutrition to support our health isn't new, but functional medicine is starting to show us that food can be a powerful tool in controlling, and even possibly reversing, chronic illness.

## HOW DOES THE AUTOIMMUNE PROTOCOL WORK?

The Autoimmune Protocol, also known as AIP, is an elimination-reintroduction diet designed to stop and reverse autoimmune disease by:

* lowering systemic inflammation in the body;
* repairing the gastrointestinal tract;
* improving digestion and nutrient absorption;
* rebalancing hormones; and
* determining food sensitivities.

The AIP diet is a functional diet that works on the core mechanisms of autoimmune illness.

## WHAT IS AN AUTOIMMUNE DISEASE?

Autoimmune disease occurs when the immune system, which is designed to protect the body from outside invaders (viruses, parasites, etc.), starts attacking itself. The human body's production of autoantibodies, immune proteins that mistakenly attack a person's own tissues, is a naturally occurring process and, under normal circumstances, the body has a system in place to clean them up and get rid of them. However, in the case of autoimmune disease, this cleanup process is broken. The autoantibodies multiply and start attacking more and more cells within the body, creating damage and corresponding physical symptoms that can't be ignored. The tissues (or organs) being attacked determine which autoimmune condition is at play. To date, over 100 autoimmune diseases have been identified and many more unidentified conditions and illnesses are suspected to be autoimmune related. Moreover, if you have one autoimmune illness, you are at a higher risk for developing another.

For an autoimmune disease to develop, a combination of factors needs to be present:

1. Genetic predisposition
2. Environmental factors (bacterial and viral infections, toxins, pollutants, chemicals, heavy metals, etc.)
3. Poor diet and lifestyle, leading to critical nutrient deficiency, gut dysbiosis (when microorganisms living in the gut are out of balance), and intestinal permeability ("leaky gut")

The science of epigenetics suggests that while we can't change our genes, it is within our power to change the expression of those genes through lifestyle and dietary modifications. Working on removing toxins and harmful chemicals from our daily lives is an important piece of the puzzle, as is addressing infections known to be linked to autoimmune disease with the help of a knowledgeable doctor. But by far the easiest and most immediate impact we can make on our health and well-being is through the food we eat (and don't eat)!

## BENEFITS OF AIP

What happens when you remove deleterious foods from your diet and start eating ones that are nutritionally dense and health promoting? First and foremost, it sets in motion a cascade of positive events in your gut. The right nutrition will repair the gut lining of the intestines and restore healthy gut microflora. This in turn will lower systemic inflammation in the body, allowing the immune system to calm down and stop producing autoantibodies. Your nutrient absorption will also improve. With these mechanisms in place, your body will be able to repair the damage caused by autoimmune disease. Your symptoms will slowly disappear, and you will enjoy a newfound energy and vitality!

Dietary and lifestyle adjustments conducive to gut health and immune regulation give your body what it needs to repair and heal on a deep, cellular level. This is what AIP is all about: healing the gut to restore proper immune function and reverse autoimmune disease.

## AIP AT A GLANCE

By now, you understand that the foods you eat (and don't eat) can repair your gut and restore proper immune function. So, let's have a closer look at what the Autoimmune Protocol entails.

The Autoimmune Protocol is comprised of two very distinct phases: the *elimination phase* and the *reintroduction phase*.

During the elimination phase, AIP removes all foods with the potential to irritate the gut as well as those that can contribute to chronic inflammation.

**WE WILL REMOVE:** Grains, gluten, dairy, eggs, beans, legumes (including soy and peanuts), nuts, seeds (including coffee and cocoa), nightshades, alcohol, processed vegetable oils, all food chemicals and additives, all refined and processed foods, and high-glycemic-load foods in excess.

I know this sounds like a lot, but remember, this phase is about more than just removing foods. It is equally important to add nutrient-dense foods to your diet to ensure your body receives the necessary building blocks to repair the damage caused by autoimmune disease.

**WE WILL ADD:** Vegetables and fruits (except nightshades), meat, poultry, organ meat, seafood, fermented foods and drinks (such as sauerkraut and kombucha), bone broth, and healthy fats.

Lifestyle factors are of equal importance during the healing phase of AIP. It is critical that you work to improve sleep, reduce stress, exercise, and maintain beneficial social connections.

Remember, the elimination phase can seem daunting, but it won't last forever. This phase of the AIP diet is temporary. During the reintroduction phase, you will begin to bring back foods that you previously eliminated.

At a minimum, you will need thirty days for the elimination phase. Three to four months is ideal, as the extended amount of time will allow your body to restore proper autoimmune response. As your body heals, you will feel your symptoms subsiding and your energy levels rebounding. You will then know it is time to begin the reintroduction phase, reincorporating eliminated foods one by one.

## DIFFERENT VERSIONS OF AIP

The Internet is full of wonderful resources on healing diets. Many, such as the Wahls Protocol by Dr. Terry Wahls, the Transition Protocol by Dr. Tom O'Bryan, the Myers Way by Dr. Amy Myers, and the Hashimoto's Protocol by Izabella Wentz, are similar to AIP. Although these related protocols may differ slightly regarding which foods to eliminate, they all rest on these common tenets:

* An overall goal of reducing inflammation and improving gut health
* Removal of inflammatory foods (gluten, dairy, grains, legumes, excess sugar)
* Removal of refined and processed foods
* Removal of food preservatives and chemicals
* A focus on whole, natural foods such as vegetables, fruits, meat, poultry, seafood, and healthy fats
* Prioritizing food variety, quality, and nutrient density

The recipes in this book follow the recommendations laid out by Dr. Sarah Ballantyne in her book *The Paleo Approach*, but most are compatible with any of these protocols. I say "most" because some protocols completely eliminate all forms of sugar, even if for a limited time. Ballantyne's Autoimmune Protocol allows one to three servings of fruit per day (about 20 grams of fructose) as well as desserts made with AIP-approved ingredients on special occasions. This makes AIP more sustainable in the long run.

# HOW TO TRANSITION YOUR DIET

It is normal to be concerned that adopting AIP will mean you won't be able to enjoy meals with your loved ones anymore. A quick look at the recipes I have created will set you at ease. You will love preparing these nourishing, tempting meals, knowing that every bite is helping your body heal and that your family will love eating them, too. Sooner than you think, AIP won't feel restrictive and will become second nature. You might even discover new foods to love!

## WHEN TO START?

I firmly believe the best time to start the Autoimmune Protocol is NOW! The sooner you begin, the sooner you will start to heal your body and feel better. There are, however, a few things to consider.

First, make sure that you have the time and the means to commit to the process once you start. Commitment and consistency are what make AIP effective. If you are going through, or are about to go through, a major life change, such as moving to a new city or starting a new job, it might be wise to postpone the start of AIP until you are settled back into a routine. Also, some people prefer to start after big holidays, especially if food plays a large role in the celebration.

## COLD TURKEY OR SLOW AND STEADY?

Faced with the challenge of starting AIP, some people will jump in and eliminate all trigger foods at once, while others prefer to take it slow, removing one food group per week, for example. The gradual approach has the advantage of breaking down the process into more manageable steps, but you will start reaping the benefits sooner by going all in. In truth, there is no wrong way to begin. The most important thing is that you take the first step and keep at it until you reach your goal.

## PREPARATION IS ESSENTIAL!

You are about to embark on an exciting journey of healing your body. Like any journey, a bit of planning goes a long way in making the adventure go smoothly. Here are some suggestions as you prepare to begin AIP:

* Have the "yes" and "no" food lists handy (see pages 18 and 19).
* Make your kitchen AIP-friendly by getting rid of everything you can no longer use.
* Plan your meals for the first week.
* Stock up on AIP-approved ingredients.
* Prepare several meals in advance and freeze them for when you don't want to cook.
* Put your support network of family and friends in place and ask for help when you need it.

# CHAPTER TWO

# WHAT CAN YOU EAT?

**DECIDING TO ADOPT** the Autoimmune Protocol is a big deal. You deserve a tremendous amount of credit for making this decision and taking your health into your own hands. That said, this is not an easy path. At times, you may feel overwhelmed by the changes you are making. Rest assured, that is completely normal. This chapter is meant to help you feel less overwhelmed. We will focus on exactly how to implement AIP—what to do, what to buy, what to avoid, and most importantly, what to eat.

I have also included detailed food lists at the end of the chapter. Make copies of these lists and keep them in your kitchen for when you are cooking, as well as in your purse or bag to pull out when grocery shopping. Adopting a new lifestyle can be tricky, but it can also be exciting. In time, what feels new and awkward will become normal and easy. Remember to keep your eye on the prize: radically improved health.

## HAPPY GUT GUIDELINES

As you navigate AIP, follow these guidelines, which are based on the recommendations of Dr. Sarah Ballantyne in *The Paleo Approach*:

1. Eat balanced meals incorporating plenty of vegetables (about three-fourths of your plate), protein (about one-fourth of your plate), and healthy fats.
2. Eat two or three large meals per day, plus a snack if you feel the need. Avoid grazing between meals or eating within two hours of bedtime.
3. Sit down to eat and chew your food slowly to facilitate digestion.
4. Eat good-quality fats from grass-fed and pasture-raised animals (such as bacon fat, lard, and tallow) and cold-pressed plant- and fruit-based oils (such as extra virgin olive oil, avocado oil, and coconut oil).
5. Eat fruit in moderation (maximum of 20 grams of fructose per day).
6. Look for the highest quality protein you can afford (grass-fed and pasture-raised animals, wild-caught seafood, and organic produce).
7. Eat as wide a variety of foods as possible to get all the nutrition you need. Prioritize seasonal produce in order to diversify your nutrient intake and reduce your grocery bill.

8. Eat organ meat! It is the most nutrient-dense part of the animal, and it's usually quite cheap to purchase. If you don't like the taste, you can "hide" it by mixing it with other ingredients (see Beginner's Liver Pâté on page 79).

9. Drink homemade bone broth regularly for its nutrient density and gut-healing properties (see Bone Broth on page 34).

10. Limit high-glycemic-load foods (such as dried fruits) to maintain good blood-sugar levels and reserve AIP treats for special occasions only.

11. Consume fermented foods (such as raw sauerkraut or lactofermented vegetables and fruits) and beverages (such as water kefir and kombucha). They contain beneficial probiotics that can help improve and regulate gut microflora.

12. Drink plenty of water to stay hydrated.

## THE AIP KITCHEN

AIP will transform not only your diet, but also your kitchen. Fresh produce, quality meats, wild-caught seafood, and healthy fats will make up the bulk of your diet, but you will also need to stock up on a few items that may be new to you. A well-stocked pantry will make your life easier and is totally worth the initial investment. These items can easily be found at your local health food store, ethnic food store, or online.

As a general rule, always read labels carefully. If a product contains food additives, preservatives, chemicals, added sugar, or any ingredient name you don't recognize, put it back on the shelf!

* *Arrowroot starch:* Used in lieu of cornstarch as a thickening agent for sauces. I also like to mix it with other denser AIP flours for a lighter texture in baked goods.

* *Baking powder:* Used to increase the volume of, and lighten the texture of, baked goods. Avoid aluminum and/or cornstarch in store-bought baking products by making your own: Mix 2 teaspoons (6 g) cream of tartar with 1 teaspoon baking soda.

* *Carob powder:* Used as a chocolate substitute. It doesn't contain any caffeine.

* *Cassava flour:* Made from peeled and ground cassava roots (or yuca/manioc). This high-fiber flour has a density similar to that of wheat flour. It's widely used for AIP baking either alone or blended with other AIP flours. Cassava flour is not interchangeable with tapioca flour in recipes, as they do not work the same way.

* *Coconut aminos:* A low-sodium alternative to soy sauce, extracted from coconut tree sap (without the coconut flavor). It's great for dressings, marinades, stir-fries, or anytime you want to add a boost of flavor to savory dishes.

* *Coconut butter:* Also known as coconut manna, this rich and creamy butter is a great alternative to nut butters. Solid at room temperature, it needs to be warmed up slowly to spread nicely.

* *Coconut flakes (unsweetened):* Great straight out of the bag for snacking. Or try toasting them with olive oil and your favorite spice for a savory, crunchy treat.
* *Coconut flour:* High-fiber flour with a rich texture and pleasant, slightly sweet taste.
* *Coconut milk (canned and unsweetened):* A rich and creamy milk widely used in AIP cuisine as a dairy-free replacement for milk and heavy cream. It's great for sauces and desserts. Look for the canned version without thickening agents or emulsifiers.
* *Coconut oil:* Nutrient-rich and easy to digest, coconut oil has a pleasant creamy texture and a light taste, which makes it a great option for cooking and baking. It's safe at higher temperatures and will turn solid at cold temperatures. Look for unrefined, cold-pressed virgin coconut oil.
* *Coconut water:* High in electrolytes, it's a good base for smoothies.
* *Collagen peptides:* A protein powder that's easy to digest and is a popular addition to smoothies and even tea. Unlike gelatin powder, this powder dissolves instantly in liquid without gelling. Look for a grass-fed, pastured-raised source.
* *Fish sauce:* Amber-colored sauce made from salted, fermented fish. Great for adding umami to savory dishes.
* *Gelatin powder (unflavored):* A protein powder that displays gelling properties when dissolved in hot liquids. It's used as an egg replacement in AIP baking and to create gelatin-based desserts and snacks, such as gummies and cheesecake. Look for a grass-fed, pasture-raised source.
* *Nutritional yeast:* This inactive yeast, in the form of yellow powder or flakes, has a distinctive nutty-cheesy flavor and is very popular for its high protein content.
* *Palm shortening:* Used in lieu of butter in baking. It is tasteless and solid at room temperature.
* *Tapioca starch:* Extracted from the crushed pulp of cassava root, this flour is used as a replacement for cornstarch to thicken sauces. It's also used in AIP baking to lighten heavier AIP flours.
* *Tapioca pearls:* Little white pearls, made of cassava, that expand and gel when mixed with a liquid. They can be used to thicken the texture of dishes or for AIP desserts.
* *Tigernut flour:* Made from small root vegetables, this grain-free, nut-free flour has a slight nutty taste and is generally used in baking.
* *Vinegars:* Apple cider vinegar, balsamic vinegar, red wine vinegar, or white wine vinegar.

# CROSS-CONTAMINATION CONCERNS

Did you know that gluten has been found to be one of the biggest culprits of leaky gut in a vast majority of autoimmune sufferers? Gluten can cross the intestinal barrier and activate an autoimmune response, setting in motion a cascade of events inside the body. It also tends to feed bad bacteria found in the gut, aggravating gut dysbiosis. For these reasons, Dr. Ballantyne recommends staying away from all foods containing gluten during and after AIP.

Unfortunately, that is easier said than done. Gluten has wormed its way into many foods, unbeknownst to the general public. From soy sauce and salad dressing to instant coffee and lunch meats, gluten can be found just about anywhere, and you will have to be vigilant with reading your labels to make sure it doesn't find its way onto your plate.

Also be aware of cross-contamination with common kitchen tools and appliances, such as toasters, wooden cutting boards, and pots used to cook pasta. The smallest particles, even crumbs and food residues, can wreak havoc in your gut.

# TIME-SAVING TECHNIQUES

You may be growing concerned thinking of all the time you will be spending in the kitchen cooking your meals. Rest assured that with a little bit of planning and organization, you will quickly learn to prepare safe and nutritious meals for yourself and your family without spending all day over the stove. It's all about making the most of the time you have.

Here are some suggestions to help:

1. Once or twice a week, sit down and plan your meals for the days ahead. Bookmark the recipes you wish to make and create a shopping list with all the ingredients you will need.
2. Immediately after grocery shopping, wash and cut your vegetables. Store washed veggies in airtight glass containers or zippered plastic bags in the refrigerator for easy access later.
3. Dedicate a time for batch cooking. Preparing several meals in advance that you can refrigerate or freeze for later is a great timesaver. Simply reheat the meals as needed.
4. If you are cooking for a family, prepare a basic meal that you can eat and then add sides for the others, such as rice, quinoa, potatoes, or gluten-free pasta.
5. Don't hesitate to ask for help from your support network. Delegate tasks such as grocery shopping and food prep. Invite a friend over to help you prepare meals.

# FOODS TO EAT

| | |
|---|---|
| VEGETABLES | artichoke, arugula, asparagus, beet, bok choy, broccoli, Brussels sprouts, butternut squash, cabbage, carrot, cauliflower, celeriac, celery, chard, collard greens, cucumber, daikon, dandelion, endive, fennel, jicama, kale, kohlrabi, leek, lettuce, mushroom, mustard greens, napa cabbage, okra, onion, parsnip, pumpkin, radicchio, radish, rhubarb, rutabaga, seaweed (such as dulse, nori, and wakame), shallot, spinach, summer squash, sweet potato, taro, turnip, water chestnuts, watercress, winter squash, yam, yuca, zucchini |
| HERBS AND SPICES | basil, bay leaf, chamomile, chives, cilantro, cinnamon, cloves, dill, fennel leaf, garlic, ginger, lavender, lemongrass, mace, marjoram, mint, oregano leaf, parsley, rosemary, saffron, sage, savory, sea salt, tarragon, thyme, turmeric, vanilla bean (but not the seeds) |
| FRUIT | apple, apricot, avocado, banana, blackberry, blueberry, cantaloupe, cherry, clementine, coconut, cranberry, date, fig, grape, grapefruit, guava, honeydew, huckleberry, kiwi, lemon, lime, mango, nectarine, olive, orange, papaya, peach, pear, persimmon, pineapple, plantain, plum, pomegranate, raspberry, strawberry, tangerine, watermelon |
| MEAT | beef, bison, chicken, duck, elk, lamb, mutton, pork, rabbit, turkey, venison, yak |
| ORGAN MEAT | bone broth, gizzard, heart, kidney, liver, tongue |
| FISH | anchovies, bass, carp, catfish, cod, haddock, halibut, herring, mackerel, mahi mahi, monkfish, salmon, sardines, snapper, sole, swordfish, tilapia, trout, tuna |
| SHELLFISH | clams, crab, crawfish, lobster, mussels, octopus, oysters, prawns, scallops, shrimp, squid |
| FERMENTS | kombucha, kvass, lactofermented fruits and vegetables, sauerkraut, water kefir |
| FATS | avocado oil, bacon fat, coconut oil, duck fat, lard (rendered pork back or kidney fat), olive oil, palm oil, palm shortening, tallow (rendered fat from beef or lamb) |
| SWEETENERS | coconut sugar, coconut syrup, dates, dried fruit, honey, maple sugar, maple syrup, molasses |
| FOODS TO CONSUME IN MODERATION | AIP treats and baked goods, coconut products, fructose (maximum 20 grams per day), green and black tea, moderate- to high-glycemic-load fruit and vegetables, natural sweeteners, salt (use mineral-rich salts) |

# FOODS TO AVOID

| | |
|---|---|
| *GRAINS* | amaranth, barley, buckwheat, bulgur, corn, farro, kamut, millet, oats, quinoa, rice, rye, sorghum, spelt, teff, wheat |
| *BEANS AND LEGUMES* | adzuki beans, black beans, black-eyed peas, calico beans, cannellini beans, chickpeas, fava beans, Great Northern beans, green beans, kidney beans, lentils, lima beans, navy beans, peanuts, peas, pinto beans, red beans, soybeans (including soy products), split peas, sugar snap peas, white beans |
| *NIGHTSHADES* | ashwagandha, bell peppers, eggplant, goji berries, ground cherries, hot peppers, potatoes, tobacco, tomatillos, tomatoes (also see spices derived from nightshades) |
| *EGGS* | chicken eggs, duck eggs, goose eggs, quail eggs |
| *DAIRY* | butter, buttermilk, butter oil, cheese, cottage cheese, cream, cream cheese, frozen yogurt, ghee, goat cheese, goat milk, ice cream, kefir, milk, sour cream, whey, whey protein, yogurt |
| *NUTS AND SEEDS* | almond, Brazil nut, cashew, chestnut, chia, cocoa, coffee, flax, hazelnut, hemp, macadamia, pecan, pine nut, pistachio, pumpkin seed, sesame seed, sunflower seed (including flours, butters, and oils derived from nuts and seeds) |
| *FATS* | canola oil, corn oil, cottonseed oil, palm kernel oil, peanut oil, safflower oil, soybean oil, sunflower oil |
| *HERBS AND SPICES* | allspice, aniseed, caraway, cardamom, cayenne pepper*, celery seed, chili pepper flakes*, chili powder*, coriander seed, cumin, curry, dill seed, fennel seed, fenugreek, juniper, mustard seed, nutmeg, paprika*, pepper (all kinds), poppy seed, red pepper flakes*, sesame seed, star anise, sumac, vanilla seeds |
| *OTHER* | alcohol, bee pollen, chlorella, emulsifiers, food additives, food chemicals, maca, NSAID medications (check with your doctor for pain management), processed sugars, processed vegetable oils, spirulina, sugar alcohol and non-nutritive sweeteners (including stevia and xylitol), thickeners |

\* Spices derived from nightshades

# ONE-WEEK MEAL PLAN

## WITH SHOPPING LIST (2 SERVINGS PER MEAL)

| | BREAKFAST | LUNCH | DINNER |
|---|---|---|---|
| SUNDAY | Fluffy Plantain Pancakes + Fruit Salad + Caffeine-Free Iced Coffee | White Minestrone + Rosemary and Thyme Focaccia | Thai Beef + Speedy Cauliflower Rice |
| MONDAY | Turkey-Veggie Breakfast Skillet | Thai Beef + Speedy Cauliflower Rice (leftovers) | Slow-Cooked Oxtail Stew |
| TUESDAY | Turkey-Veggie Breakfast Skillet (leftovers) | White Minestrone + Rosemary and Thyme Focaccia (leftovers) | Slow-Cooked Oxtail Stew (leftovers) |
| WEDNESDAY | Maple-Bacon Patties + Baked Spaghetti Squash | Slow-Cooked Oxtail Stew (leftovers) | Baby Arugula and Root Vegetable Salad + Rustic Meatloaf |
| THURSDAY | Maple-Bacon Patties + Baked Spaghetti Squash (leftovers) | Baby Arugula and Root Vegetable Salad + Rustic Meatloaf (leftovers) | Tex-Mex Marinated Steak + Antioxidant Kale Salad |
| FRIDAY | Express Cauliflower "Oatmeal" + Chicken-Apple Patties | Tex-Mex Marinated Steak + Antioxidant Kale Salad (leftovers) | Nourishing Seafood Gratin |
| SATURDAY | Express Cauliflower "Oatmeal" + Chicken-Apple Patties (leftovers) + Pumpkin Spice Latte | Rainbow Veggie Wraps + Lime–Sea Salt Tostones | Nourishing Seafood Gratin (leftovers) |

*The Autoimmune Protocol Made Simple Cookbook*

## MEAT

* 14 ounces (395 g) uncooked bacon + 6 cooked slices
* 1 pound (450 g) ground beef
* 1¼ pounds (560 g) beef flank steak
* 1 pound (450 g) beef skirt steak
* 1 pound (450 g) ground chicken
* 1½ quarts (1.5 L) + 3⅓ cups (800 ml) chicken bone broth (page 34)
* 4 pounds (1.8 kg) oxtail
* 2 pounds (900 g) ground pork
* 1 pound (450 g) ground turkey

## SEAFOOD

* 1 pound (450 g) skinless cod fillets

## FRESH PRODUCE

* 3 apricots
* 3 avocados
* 4 ounces (115 g) baby arugula
* 2 cups (200 g) riced broccoli (page 89)
* 1 pound (450 g) butternut squash
* 2¼ pounds (1 kg) + ⅔ cup (70 g) shredded carrots
* 2 pounds (900 g) cauliflower
* 4 cups (400 g) riced cauliflower (page 89)
* 4 chard leaves
* 12 ounces (340 g) cherries
* 4 collard green leaves
* 2 1-inch (2.5 cm) knobs fresh ginger + ½ teaspoon grated
* 1 green plantain
* 5 ounces (150 g) kale
* 12 ounces (340 g) leeks
* 1 lemon
* Zest and juice of 2 limes

* 8 ounces (225 g) + 3 ounces (85 g) white button or portobello mushrooms
* 1 orange
* 3 pounds (1.4 kg) parsnips
* 1 peach
* 10 radishes
* 3 cups (270 g) sliced red cabbage
* 8 ounces (225 g) red onions + ⅓ cup (50 g) minced
* 1 ripe plantain
* 7 scallions
* 1 shallot + ⅓ cup (50 g) minced
* 6 ounces (170 g) shiitake mushrooms
* 2½ to 3 pounds (1.1 to 1.4 kg) spaghetti squash
* 8 ounces (225 g) strawberries
* 1½ pounds (675 g) sweet potatoes + 2 cups (270 g) shredded
* 1½ pounds (675 g) yellow onions + 1½ cups (240 g) chopped

## HERBS AND SPICES

* For garnishes: fresh basil, mint, thyme, scallion, cilantro, parsley
* 2 bay leaves
* 1 tablespoon (5 g) roasted chicory root
* 1 teaspoon dried cilantro
* ½ teaspoon ground cinnamon
* 1⅔ cups (26 g) chopped fresh cilantro
* 2 tablespoons (15 g) dandelion root
* 7 cloves garlic
* ¾ teaspoon garlic powder
* 1 tablespoon (2 g) + ½ teaspoon dried marjoram
* 1 teaspoon onion flakes

* ½ tablespoon (3 g) + 1 teaspoon dried oregano
* 1½ tablespoons (4 g) fresh oregano
* ¾ cup (45 g) minced fresh parsley
* 1½ teaspoons (2 g) dried rosemary
* 1 teaspoon dried sage
* 8 Thai basil leaves
* 1 teaspoon dried thyme
* 1 vanilla bean

## PANTRY ITEMS

* 1 (¼-ounce, or 7 g) packet active dry yeast
* 2 tablespoons (30 ml) apple cider vinegar
* 3 tablespoons (24 g) arrowroot flour
* ¼ teaspoon baking powder
* 1 cup (140 g) cassava flour
* ½ cup (120 ml) coconut aminos
* 1 cup (240 ml) coconut cream
* ½ cup + 3 tablespoons (80 g) coconut flour
* ½ cup (120 ml) coconut oil
* ⅓ cup + 9 tablespoons (210 ml) extra virgin olive oil
* 1 tablespoon (15 ml) fish sauce
* 2 (14-ounce, or 400 ml) cans + 2½ cups (600 ml) + ⅓ cup (80 ml) full-fat coconut milk
* 2 teaspoons (6 g) gelatin powder
* ½ tablespoon (8 ml) honey
* 3 tablespoons + 3 teaspoons (60 ml) maple syrup
* ¼ cup (60 ml) palm shortening
* 3 tablespoons (50 g) pumpkin puree
* 4 sheets nori

# CHAPTER THREE

# HOW TO REINTRODUCE FOODS

**AS YOUR BODY HEALS** and you begin feeling measurably better, you can start reintroducing foods into your diet, one by one, monitoring yourself for symptoms. This reintroduction process will help you determine your own food intolerances, which in turn will allow you to tailor your diet to meet your own personal needs and preferences.

Does this mean that you will go back to eating like you did before beginning AIP? No. While the ultimate goal of the reintroduction process is to widen your diet as much as possible, in order to maintain optimal health, you will have to stay away from all foods harmful to the gut. For instance, Dr. Sarah Ballantyne recommends staying away from gluten and soy forever. She further recommends avoiding processed sugar, refined vegetable oils, food additives, and in general, all foods poor in nutrients. Once your symptoms are fully under control and you have successfully introduced many nutrient-dense foods, you may be able to occasionally eat other things. Certain gluten-free grains, such as rice and organic corn, for instance, as well as soaked and sprouted legumes, can be welcome additions to your diet provided they do not exacerbate your autoimmune condition.

Only you will know how strict you need to be to maintain a level of good health. This phase is about experimenting. Remember, you always have the option of reverting to the elimination phase should your symptoms creep up once again.

## STARTING REINTRODUCTIONS

There is no universal rule as to when you should start reintroducing foods. The timing depends on how long it will take your body to return to a level of good health, and on this we are all different.

Dr. Ballantyne recommends a bare minimum of 30 days on AIP, though many people opt to remain in the elimination phase longer. At the very least, wait until your gut has sufficiently healed before attempting any reintroductions. You will know that your gut is functioning properly when you can digest your food well without gastrointestinal distress, your autoimmune disease is no longer active, and your symptoms have subsided.

Give your body time to heal and avoid rushing the process. It will be worth the wait! Know that the longer you wait, the more resilient your body becomes, increasing the chances of successful reintroductions.

The lifestyle aspect of the Autoimmune Protocol also influences how you will react to a reintroduced food. More than ever, make sure your stress is under control, you are sleeping well, you are exercising, and if possible, you are spending time in nature. When these elements are in balance, your body will more easily tolerate the reintroduction of new foods, which of course is the goal.

# HOW TO REINTRODUCE FOODS

The reintroduction process, also called *food challenge*, may seem slow and meticulous, but it is important to follow the steps in order to detect not only strong, fast-appearing food reactions, but also the more insidious ones that may crop up after several days. Remember, slow and steady wins the race!

Reactions will usually appear within 1 to 4 hours after eating the offending food, with symptoms culminating within 24 hours. In some cases, it may take up to 3 to 7 days for a reaction to surface. If you notice any symptom at any time during the food challenge, stop immediately and wait until your symptoms have completely subsided before trying again.

It is a good idea to keep a daily food journal as you navigate the reintroduction process. Jotting down what you eat, when you eat it, and if you notice any change at all in how you feel, including physical symptoms and mood fluctuations, will help you identify patterns between the food you eat and the reactions you experience.

## FOOD CHALLENGE PROCEDURE

* **STEP 1:** Choose a food to reintroduce. Eat ½ teaspoon and wait 15 minutes. If symptoms appear, stop.
* **STEP 2:** If no symptoms appear, eat 1 full teaspoon and wait another 15 minutes. If symptoms appear, stop.
* **STEP 3:** If no symptoms appear, eat 1½ teaspoons and wait 2 to 3 hours. If symptoms appear, stop.
* **STEP 4:** If no symptoms appear, eat a normal-size portion and wait 3 days (up to 7 days if you are particularly sensitive and react easily to many foods). During this period, do not eat more of the food you challenged and do not eat any other new food. If symptoms appear, stop. If no symptoms appear, congratulations! This food is now potentially safe for you to eat.

When reintroducing spices, prepare a dish and season generously with the spice you are challenging. Follow the standard procedure, starting with one small bite, then two bites, and then three bites, before eating a normal-size portion.

When reintroducing alcoholic beverages, drink a small serving (8–9 ounces [230–260 ml] of gluten-free beer or cider, 5 ounces [145 ml] of wine, 3–4 ounces [85–120 ml] of fortified wine, 2–3 ounces [60–85 ml] of liqueur, or 1–1½ ounces [30–45 ml] spirits), and then wait 1 week before having another serving, watching for symptoms. Do not exceed two servings of alcohol per week if you have an autoimmune disease.

## ORDER OF REINTRODUCTIONS

There are two schools of thought on the order of reintroductions. One theory is to let your cravings guide you. You might very well decide to start with chocolate or coffee, for example, just because you miss it the most. The other theory, which is suggested by Dr. Ballantyne, prioritizes the foods that have the highest nutritional value and the least likelihood of triggering an autoimmune response.

The following is the order of reintroductions as suggested by Dr. Ballantyne. Which food should *you* choose first to reintroduce into your diet? Once again, there isn't a general rule here. Dr. Ballantyne's stages are simply templates—the ultimate decision is up to you.

* **STEP 1:** egg yolks, fresh legumes (such as peas and green beans), fruit-based spices, seed-based spices, seed and nut oils, grass-fed ghee
* **STEP 2:** seeds, nuts (except cashews and pistachios), cocoa or chocolate, egg whites, grass-fed butter, alcohol in small quantities
* **STEP 3:** cashews and pistachios, eggplant, bell peppers, paprika, coffee, grass-fed raw cream, fermented grass-fed dairy (such as yogurt and kefir)
* **STEP 4:** grass-fed whole milk, grass-fed cheese, chile peppers, tomatoes, potatoes, nightshade spices, alcohol in larger quantities, white rice, soaked and sprouted legumes, soaked and sprouted gluten-free grains, any other food you used to be allergic to* before AIP

* Please keep in mind that those with life-threatening allergies should never attempt to consume that which they are allergic to unless under the express care of a doctor, and those with celiac disease should never knowingly consume gluten.

# MANAGING EXPECTATIONS

Ideally, during a food challenge, no symptoms appear and you can incorporate that food back into your general diet. Enjoy this small victory! Be aware, however, that some food reactions, undetectable at first, may increase as you start eating this new food regularly, perhaps on a daily basis. In such situations, stop eating the offending food and give it another try at a later date.

That said, a reaction might occur. Reactions can range anywhere from mild to severe and encompass physical as well as psychological manifestations. Potential symptoms include:

* resurgence of the symptoms of your autoimmune disease;
* gastrointestinal disturbances such as pain, gas, bloating, constipation, or diarrhea;
* sudden fatigue and lack of energy;

* food cravings;
* sleep disturbances;
* headaches;
* brain fog;
* increased mucus production and the need to clear your throat;
* itchy and watery eyes;
* skin rashes;
* aches and pains; and
* mood swings, such as anxiety or feeling depressed.

Although experiencing a reaction can be disheartening, remember that it is not the end of everything. If you react strongly to a food, stop eating it immediately and allow your body to heal. You can always try to introduce the food again later as your gut health improves.

## HANDLING FLARE-UPS

Remember that an autoimmune flare-up triggered by a food reintroduction will be temporary. When you stop eating the offending food, your symptoms will fade rapidly. In the meantime, be gentle with yourself and increase your self-care. Below are some suggestions to help you get through the flare-up and quickly get back on track.

1. Slow down as much as you can.
2. Relieve pain if you need to.
3. Prioritize your sleep.
4. Increase your intake of healing foods, such as bone broth, organ meat, and turmeric.
5. Destress and detoxify with an Epsom salts bath.
6. Keep your body moving with gentle exercise.
7. Do all the things that make you happy!

Reintroducing foods is an exciting time, but it is a *process*. Take your time. Your body will thank you for it!

# RECIPE INDEX

## HOMEMADE BASICS AND STAPLES

* Onion-Basil Crackers
* Rosemary and Thyme Focaccia
* No-Fail Turmeric Tortillas
* Bone Broth
* Dairy-Free Vanilla-Maple Creamer
* Strawberry-Beet Salsa
* Nightshade-Free Italian Sauce
* Mayonnaise
* "Cheesy" Sauce
* Spicy Guacamole
* Garlic-Lemon Mayonnaise
* Chimichurri Verde
* Ranch Dressing
* Creamy Cilantro Dressing
* Shallot Vinaigrette
* Citrus Vinaigrette

## BREAKFASTS

* Fluffy Plantain Pancakes
* Grain-Free & Nut-Free Granola
* Express Cauliflower "Oatmeal"
* Caffeine-Free Iced Coffee
* Pumpkin Spice Latte
* Hidden Veggies Smoothie
* Carrot Cake Smoothie
* Pork-Veggie Breakfast Skillet
* Turkey-Veggie Breakfast Skillet
* Loaded Sweet Potatoes
* Chicken-Apple Patties
* Maple-Bacon Patties

## SMALL BITES

* Chicken-Veggie Poppers
* Lime–Sea Salt Tostones
* AIP Nachos
* Cheesy Bacon Sweet Potato Sliders
* Garlic Refrigerator Pickles
* Roasted Fennel Hummus
* Rainbow Veggie Wraps
* Cocktail Cheese Bites
* Dairy-Free Zucchini Cheese
* Beginner's Liver Pâté
* Curry Chicken Salad
* Mediterranean Tuna Salad

## SOUPS AND SALADS

* Dandelion-Zoodle Salad
* Jicama-Mango Salad
* Refreshing Cauli-Tabbouleh
* Antioxidant Kale Salad
* Mixed Veggie Bowl
* Baby Arugula and Root Vegetable Salad
* Turmeric-Ginger Soup
* Julienne Vegetable Soup
* Lemongrass Chicken Soup
* White Minestrone
* Cream of Parsnip Soup
* Rustic Chard and Bacon Soup

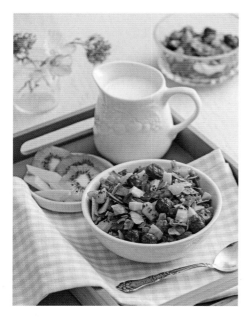

## VEGETABLES

* Baked Spaghetti Squash
* Crispy Yuca Fries
* Roasted Root Vegetables and Citrus
* Speedy Cauliflower Rice
* Creamy Mashed Broccoli
* Coleslaw
* Veggie Tacos
* Creamed Kale
* Vegetable Curry
* Sweet Potato Gratin
* Basil Zucchini Noodles
* Simple Roasted Turnips

## MEAT-BASED MAIN DISHES

* Tex-Mex Marinated Steak
* Honey-Lime Chicken with Peach Salsa
* Meatballs
* Tacos for the Meat Lover
* Versatile Pulled Pork Carnitas
* Beef-Bison Burgers
* Thai Beef
* Rustic Meatloaf
* Beef Liver Skillet
* One-Pot Chicken Bake
* Slow-Cooked Oxtail Stew
* Slow-Cooked Plum Chicken Stew

## SEAFOOD

* Truffle Salt Sea Scallops
* Pan-Fried Fish Sticks
* Seafood Chowder
* Seared Tuna Tataki
* Smoked Salmon and Fennel Salad
* Salmon Poke Bowl
* Coconut Milk Shrimp Ceviche
* Garlic-Seaweed Shrimp
* Baked Cod "En Papillote"
* Nourishing Seafood Gratin
* Fish Tacos
* Quick Tuna Tartare

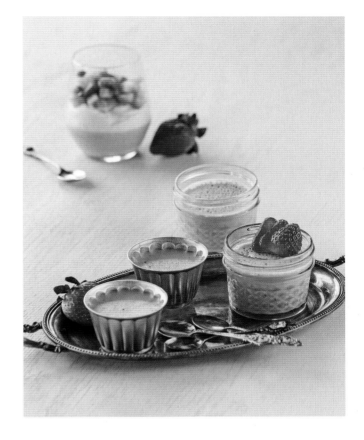

## DESSERTS AND DRINKS

* Fruit Salad with Coconut Whipped Cream
* Gut-Healing Turmeric Gummies
* Vanilla-Strawberry Ice Cream
* Strawberry-Lime Mousse
* Tummy-Soothing Popsicles
* Tapioca Pudding with Peach-Lavender Compote
* Coconut-Berry Trifle
* Mini Raspberry Cheesecakes
* Delectable Cherry Crumble
* Citrus-Rosemary Spritzer
* Hibiscus-Lavender Lemonade
* AIP Mule

# CHAPTER FOUR

# HOMEMADE BASICS AND STAPLES

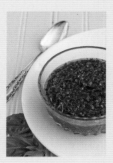

**ANYTHING BUT BORING,** cooking basics—from salad dressing to bone broth—are the backbone of any kitchen. This chapter is chock-full of indispensable recipes you will use again and again when preparing meals.

With its focus on therapeutic and anti-inflammatory foods, AIP can seem austere to the untrained eye. In truth, AIP utilizes staples such as marinades and sauces to enhance the appeal of many otherwise unadorned recipes. To make your cooking mouthwatering, I recommend adding as many of these little beauties to your repertoire as possible.

I strongly recommend batch cooking, which is a wonderful timesaver. First things first: Plan your meals in advance. It makes all the difference. Who wants to look at the clock at 5:45 p.m. and realize there's no plan for dinner? Plan at least four to five dinners ahead. Write them down (there's no need to be fancy; a few notes will do), shop, and prepare anything that can be stored in the fridge for a few days, such as sauces and marinades, ahead of time. Having those extra sauces, for example, at hand means you can use them to dress salads, garnish vegetables, and give a second life to leftovers.

Finally, you may be wondering about that illustrious bone broth everyone is raving about. Don't worry. I've got you covered. This kitchen staple is widely used in the Autoimmune Protocol in soups, sauces, and even vegetable dishes. Either on its own as a restorative "cuppa" or as a base to a hearty stew, my bone broth will have you on the road to health in no time.

Welcome to AIP Homemade Basics and Staples.

# ONION-BASIL CRACKERS

ONE OF THE CHALLENGES OF AIP IS FINDING A SATISFYINGLY CRISP CRACKER. ALMOST ALL CRACKERS ARE MADE WITH WHEAT OR RICE, BOTH OF WHICH ARE VERBOTEN. BUT SOMETIMES, WE JUST REALLY NEED SOMETHING CRUNCHY WITH WHICH TO SCOOP DIP, HUMMUS, OR LIVER PÂTÉ. THESE SAVORY CRACKERS DO THE JOB AND THEN SOME! FEEL FREE TO TRY MAKING THEM WITH YOUR FAVORITE DRIED HERBS.

## directions

1. Place the oven rack in the top third position and preheat the oven to 400°F (200°C). Line 2 baking sheets with parchment paper.

2. Mix the cassava flour, tigernut flour, basil, onion flakes, and sea salt in a large bowl with a spatula. Add the water and olive oil. Mix until you obtain a soft dough.

3. Scoop out ½ tablespoon (8 g) of dough and roll it into a small ball with your hands. Place the ball on the prepared baking sheet, cover it with a small piece of parchment paper, and flatten it to about ⅛ inch (3 mm) thick or 2 inches (5 cm) wide using the bottom of a measuring cup. Repeat with the rest of the dough, arranging about 15 crackers on each baking sheet.

4. Bake for 13 to 15 minutes, until the edges of the crackers start to turn brown. Transfer to a wire rack to cool completely.

## ingredients

½ cup (70 g) cassava flour

½ cup (60 g) tigernut flour

2 teaspoons (1.5 g) dried basil

1 teaspoon onion flakes

¾ teaspoon fine sea salt

½ cup (120 ml) water

2 tablespoons (30 ml) extra virgin olive oil

### prep time
15 minutes

### cook time
15 minutes

### yield
30 crackers

## note

STORE CRACKERS FOR UP TO 7 DAYS AT ROOM TEMPERATURE IN AN AIRTIGHT CONTAINER TO PRESERVE THEIR CRISPINESS.

*note*

THIS FOCACCIA WILL
KEEP, WRAPPED IN A
KITCHEN TOWEL AND
STORED IN A COOL,
DRY PLACE, FOR UP TO
5 DAYS.

# ROSEMARY AND THYME FOCACCIA

AH, THE JOY OF DIPPING A FRAGRANT PIECE OF BREAD INTO SOMETHING DELICIOUS! THIS SOFT AND AROMATIC FOCACCIA IS DIVINE WHEN PAIRED WITH SO MANY THINGS. ITS TENDER TEXTURE MAKES IT A FAVORITE FOR DIPPING IN A LITTLE BIT OF OLIVE OIL AND DRIED HERBS, LIKE THE ITALIANS DO. IT WILL TASTE EVEN BETTER IF YOU BREAK IT APART INTO SMALL PIECES INSTEAD OF SLICING IT. YOU MAY ALSO TRY IT WITH A LIGHT SOUP, A HEARTY STEW, OR A SPOONFUL OF LIVER PÂTÉ.

## directions

1. Line a baking sheet with parchment paper.

2. Combine ¼ cup (60 ml) of the warm water with the maple syrup in a small bowl. Add the yeast and stir. Wait about 5 minutes for the mixture to start foaming. (If the yeast doesn't foam, throw it away and start over.)

3. Meanwhile, combine the cassava flour, coconut flour, rosemary, thyme, and sea salt in a large bowl. Mix well with a spatula and form a well in the middle. Carefully pour the remaining ¾ cup (180 ml) warm water and palm shortening into the well. Add the yeast mixture. Mix well with a spatula until the dough is smooth. Knead 8 to 10 times with your hands and form the dough into a ball.

4. Transfer the dough to the parchment-lined baking sheet. Flatten it with your hands to form a 1-inch (2.5 cm)-thick loaf. Cover with a light kitchen towel and let rest in a warm place for 30 minutes.

5. Place the oven rack in the middle position and preheat the oven to 400°F (200°C).

6. After 30 minutes, uncover the dough (don't knead it again!) and score it 3 times at an angle with a serrated knife. Sprinkle with more rosemary and thyme.

7. Bake for about 35 minutes, until the bread turns golden. Transfer to a wire rack and let cool completely before eating.

## ingredients

1 cup (240 ml) warm (110°F to 115°F [43 to 46°C]) water, divided

1 teaspoon maple syrup

1 (¼-ounce, or 7 g) packet active dry yeast

1 cup (140 g) cassava flour

½ cup (56 g) coconut flour

1½ teaspoons (2 g) minced dried rosemary, plus extra for garnish

1 teaspoon dried thyme, plus extra for garnish

¾ teaspoon fine sea salt

¼ cup (60 ml) melted palm shortening

## prep time
40 minutes

## cook time
35 minutes

## yield
1 (14-ounce, or 392 g) focaccia

# NO-FAIL TURMERIC TORTILLAS

## ingredients

1 cup (140 g) cassava flour

1 tablespoon (9 g) coconut flour

¾ teaspoon fine sea salt

½ teaspoon baking powder

½ teaspoon turmeric powder

⅔ cup (160 ml) warm water

3 tablespoons (45 ml) extra virgin olive oil

½ teaspoon apple cider vinegar

## prep time
10 minutes

## cook time
25 minutes

## yield
6 tortillas

TORTILLAS ARE PERFECT FOR WRAPS AND TACOS, BUT AIP-FRIENDLY VERSIONS CAN BE HARD TO FIND. THESE SOFT AND DELICATELY PERFUMED TORTILLAS SOLVE THAT PROBLEM IN A SNAP. I LIKE TO DOUBLE THE INGREDIENTS AND MAKE A BIG BATCH, FREEZING SOME FOR LATER. AND DON'T WORRY IF YOU CAN'T SHAPE THEM PERFECTLY—YOU GET POINTS FOR TRYING! IF YOU DON'T HAVE A ROLLING PIN HANDY, A TALL GLASS WILL DO THE TRICK.

## directions

1. Combine the cassava flour, coconut flour, sea salt, baking powder, and turmeric powder in a large bowl. In a separate bowl, stir together the water, olive oil, and apple cider vinegar.

2. Pour the liquid mixture into the dry ingredients. Mix with a spatula to roughly combine the ingredients. Knead a few times with your hands until a smooth dough forms.

3. Divide the dough in half. Divide each half into 3 equal portions, forming a total of 6 little dough balls. Roll each ball between 2 sheets of parchment paper with a rolling pin to form a thin, round circle about 6 inches (15 cm) in diameter. As you stack the rolled-out tortillas, insert a piece of parchment paper between each layer so they don't stick together.

4. Heat a nonstick skillet over medium-high heat. Cook each tortilla, uncovered, for about 2 minutes, until the bottom shows little golden spots and bubbles form on the surface. Flip with a spatula and cook for an additional 1½ to 2 minutes.

5. Serve warm, refrigerate, or freeze for later use.

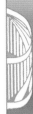

# BONE BROTH

BONE BROTH IS AN ESSENTIAL PART OF THE AUTOIMMUNE PROTOCOL FOR ITS NUTRIENT DENSITY AND GUT-HEALING PROPERTIES. COLLAGEN, RELEASED DURING THE SIMMERING PROCESS, PLAYS A KEY ROLE IN RESTORING THE INTEGRITY OF THE GUT LINING AND SUPPORTS A HEALTHY DIGESTIVE TRACT. SIP A CUP EVERY DAY OR USE IT TO PREPARE NUTRITIOUS MEALS SUCH AS SOUPS, STEWS, AND SAUCES.

## *ingredients*

2½ to 3 pounds
(1.1 to 1.4 kg) bones
from chicken, beef, lamb,
pork, etc.

3 quarts (2.8 L) water

1 tablespoon (15 ml)
apple cider vinegar

## *prep time*
5 minutes

## *cook time*
8 to 24 hours

## *yield*
3 quarts (2.8 L)

## *directions*

1. Place the bones, water, and apple cider vinegar in a 6-quart (5.4-L) slow cooker. (The water should entirely cover the bones.) Cover securely and simmer on low for 8 to 24 hours.

2. Discard the bones and pour the liquid through a strainer to catch any small bits and pieces.

3. Serve or save for later use by letting the bone broth cool and transferring to sealed glass containers. Store refrigerated.

## *notes*

ADD A FEW CHICKEN FEET FOR A BROTH THAT WILL GEL EVERY TIME, THUS INCREASING ITS GUT-HEALING GELATIN CONTENT. GELATIN IS ALSO GOOD FOR YOUR SKIN AND HAIR.

DON'T MIND IF THERE'S A LITTLE MEAT ON THE BONES; IT WILL GIVE THE BROTH AN EXTRA BOOST OF FLAVOR.

BONE BROTH WILL KEEP FOR UP TO 1 WEEK IN THE REFRIGERATOR, AND IT ALSO FREEZES WELL. TO FREEZE, ALLOW THE BROTH TO COOL COMPLETELY AT ROOM TEMPERATURE. TRANSFER TO A TALL GLASS CONTAINER AND CLOSE THE LID TIGHTLY. STORE IN THE FREEZER FOR UP TO 6 MONTHS.

# DAIRY-FREE VANILLA-MAPLE CREAMER

THIS DELICIOUS DAIRY-FREE CREAMER IS ABSOLUTELY THE BEST TO LIGHTEN YOUR HERBAL COFFEE OR TEA. WHEN REFRIGERATED, IT CAN THICKEN A BIT, SO EITHER SCOOP A SPOONFUL OR TWO DIRECTLY INTO YOUR HOT HERBAL COFFEE OR TEA OR WARM IT UP A BIT SO IT CAN REGAIN ITS LIQUID CONSISTENCY.

## directions

1. Place the coconut milk, maple syrup, and vanilla bean in a small saucepan. Bring the mixture to a boil over high heat, stirring constantly with a spoon or a whisk. Reduce the heat to medium-low and let simmer for 20 minutes.

2. Discard the vanilla bean. Allow the creamer to cool to room temperature. Store in a glass bottle with a lid and refrigerate until needed.

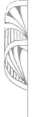

## note

THIS RECIPE REQUIRES A VANILLA BEAN. VANILLA BEANS ARE AIP COMPLIANT, BUT THE SEEDS INSIDE THE BEAN AREN'T PART OF THE ELIMINATION PHASE. EITHER USE THE BEAN WHOLE OR IF YOU CUT IT OPEN, SCRAPE OUT ALL OF THE SEEDS AND DISCARD.

## ingredients

1 (14-ounce, or 400 ml) can full-fat coconut milk

2 tablespoons (30 ml) maple syrup

1 vanilla bean

## prep time
5 minutes

## cook time
20 minutes

## yield
1 ¾ cups (420 ml)

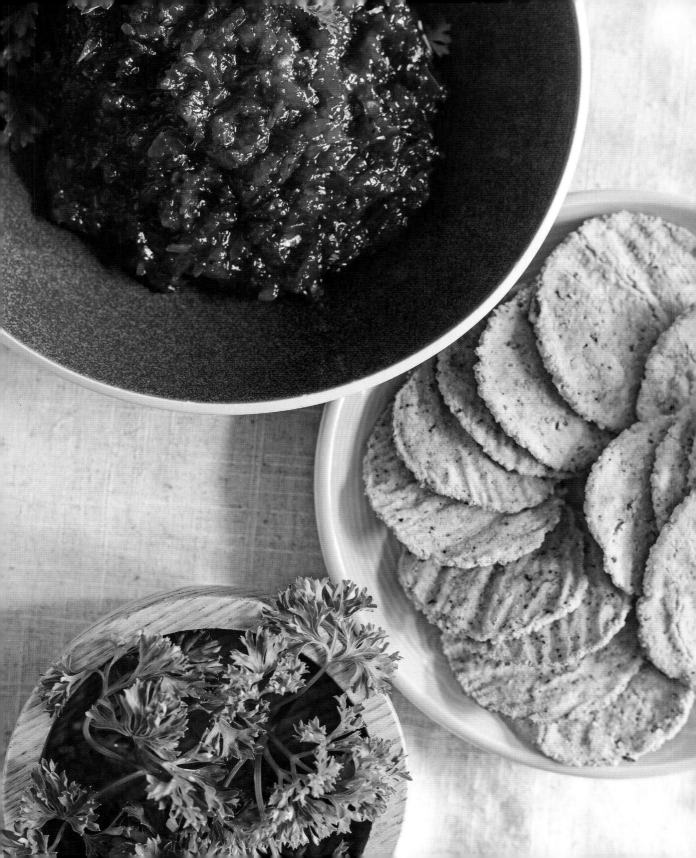

# STRAWBERRY-BEET SALSA

THIS ONE-OF-A-KIND SALSA WILL KNOCK YOUR SOCKS OFF WITH ITS TART FLAVOR AND VIBRANT COLOR! I LIKE MY SALSA ON THE CHUNKY SIDE, BUT FEEL FREE TO MIX IT UNTIL SMOOTH AND CREAMY. BEETS CAN TAKE A WHILE TO COOK, SO TO SAVE TIME, I USUALLY COOK THEM THE DAY BEFORE I MAKE THIS SALSA, WHILE I'M TENDING TO OTHER TASKS. WITH PRECOOKED BEETS, I CAN PUT IT TOGETHER IN LITTLE TIME.

## directions

1. Combine all the ingredients in a food processor and mix until you obtain the desired consistency: chunky or smooth. Scrape down the sides of the bowl with a spatula as needed.

2. Chill in the refrigerator and serve.

## ingredients

8 ounces (225 g) cooked beets, peeled and diced

8 ounces (225 g) fresh strawberries, hulled and quartered

4 ounces (112 g) red onion, chopped

½ packed cup (30 g) chopped fresh parsley

1½ tablespoons (22 ml) lemon juice

¾ teaspoon fine sea salt

## prep time
10 minutes

## yield
2½ cups (600 g)

## notes

SERVE THIS SALSA WITH AN ASSORTMENT OF CUT VEGETABLES (SUCH AS CARROTS, SLICED RADISHES, OR CAULIFLOWER FLORETS), TO PREPARE RAINBOW VEGGIE WRAPS (PAGE 74), IN TACOS, OR TO BRIGHTEN UP ANY SALAD. IT ALSO GOES GREAT ON ONION-BASIL CRACKERS (PAGE 29).

WILL KEEP IN THE REFRIGERATOR FOR UP TO 5 DAYS

## NIGHTSHADE-FREE ITALIAN SAUCE

TOMATO SAUCE IS A NO-NO ON AIP, BUT SOME MEALS—LIKE MEATBALLS—SIMPLY SCREAM FOR A BIG, BOLD RED SAUCE. FOR THE TIMES WHEN YOU SIMPLY MUST HAVE TOMATO SAUCE, TRY THIS HEARTY "NO TOMATO" RED SAUCE. YOU WON'T MISS WHAT'S NOT THERE, I PROMISE!

### *ingredients*

1 (15-ounce, or 420 g) can butternut squash puree

8 ounces (225 g) cooked red beets, peeled and chopped

3 tablespoons (45 ml) full-fat coconut milk

1 tablespoon (15 ml) apple cider vinegar

1 tablespoon (15 ml) coconut aminos

2 teaspoons (1.5 g) dried basil

2 teaspoons (1 g) dried marjoram

1½ teaspoons (9 g) fine sea salt

1 teaspoon onion powder

1 teaspoon dried oregano

*prep time*
8 minutes

*yield*
3 cups (700 ml)

### *directions*

1. Combine all the ingredients in a blender or food processor. Blend on high for about 30 seconds, until you obtain a smooth and creamy sauce. Check the seasoning and adjust the salt to taste.

2. Store in a glass container and refrigerate until needed. Reheat on the stovetop over low heat, stirring frequently.

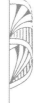

### *note*

THE SAUCE WILL KEEP, COVERED, IN THE REFRIGERATOR FOR UP TO 5 DAYS. IT FREEZES WELL. SERVE WITH MEATBALLS (PAGE 123), BASIL ZUCCHINI NOODLES (PAGE 116), OR RUSTIC MEATLOAF (PAGE 130).

## MAYONNAISE

TRADITIONALLY MADE WITH EGGS, PEOPLE EITHER LOVE OR HATE MAYONNAISE. IF YOU ARE A FAN, THIS AIP-FRIENDLY MAYO IS THE ANSWER TO YOUR "I CAN'T EAT REAL MAYONNAISE" CONUNDRUM.

### *ingredients*

⅓ cup (80 ml) avocado oil

⅓ cup (80 ml) extra virgin olive oil

⅓ cup (80 ml) palm shortening

1 teaspoon lemon juice

Pinch of fine sea salt

*prep time*
5 minutes

*yield*
1 cup (240 ml)

### *directions*

1. Combine all the ingredients in a large mixing bowl and beat with a hand mixer for about 30 seconds, until you obtain a smooth and creamy texture. Check the seasoning and adjust the salt and lemon to taste.

2. Store in an airtight container in the refrigerator. For a creamier consistency, remove from the refrigerator 20 minutes before serving.

### *note*

MAYONNAISE WILL KEEP IN THE REFRIGERATOR FOR UP TO 7 DAYS.

# "CHEESY" SAUCE

WHAT'S THAT? YOU THOUGHT CHEESE WAS OUT ON AIP!? WELL, IT IS. THIS VERSATILE SAUCE HAS A SECRET INGREDIENT: NUTRITIONAL YEAST. THIS INACTIVE FORM OF YEAST ADDS A BOOST OF UMAMI AND CAN BE USED TO REPLACE CHEESE IN MANY RECIPES. ALSO TRY IT SPRINKLED ON COOKED VEGETABLES OR BAKED ONTO AIP FOCACCIA.

## directions

1. Place the cauliflower rice and bone broth in a saucepan. Bring to a boil over high heat. Reduce the heat to medium and cook, stirring a few times, for about 8 minutes, until tender.

2. Transfer the cauliflower rice mixture to a high-speed blender. Add the nutritional yeast and sea salt. Blend on high for about 30 seconds, until smooth and creamy.

3. Check the seasoning and adjust the salt to taste. Serve immediately or let cool and refrigerate until needed.

*note*

"CHEESY" SAUCE WILL KEEP IN A GLASS CONTAINER, COVERED, IN THE REFRIGERATOR FOR UP TO 7 DAYS.

*ingredients*

2 cups (235 g) raw Cauliflower Rice (page 106)

1 cup (240 ml) Bone Broth (page 34)

2 tablespoons (16 g) nutritional yeast

½ teaspoon fine sea salt

*prep time*
10 minutes

*cook time*
8 minutes

*yield*
1½ cups (350 ml)

---

# SPICY GUACAMOLE

THIS GUAC GOES WITH EVERYTHING. FRESH GINGER (A POWERFUL ANTI-INFLAMMATORY AND NATURAL IMMUNE BOOSTER), LIME JUICE, AND ONIONS COME TOGETHER TO CREATE AN UPLIFTING, HOT AND SPICY COMBO. ENJOY IT AS A DIP, ON TACOS, OR AS A SANDWICH SPREAD.

## directions

1. Combine all the ingredients in a bowl and mix thoroughly.

2. Chill in the refrigerator until needed. Serve the same day.

*note*

IF YOU PREPARE THIS GUACAMOLE AHEAD OF TIME, SPRINKLE WITH LIME JUICE AND THEN SEAL WITH A PIECE OF PLASTIC WRAP DIRECTLY ON TOP TO PREVENT BROWNING.

*ingredients*

2 large avocados, peeled, pitted, and mashed

⅓ cup (6 g) chopped cilantro

⅓ cup (50 g) minced red onion

2 tablespoons (30 ml) freshly squeezed lime juice

1 (1-inch, or 2.5 cm) knob fresh ginger, peeled and grated

¼ teaspoon fine sea salt

¼ teaspoon garlic powder

*prep time*
12 minutes

*yield*
1 cup (240 ml)

*Homemade Basics and Staples*

# GARLIC-LEMON MAYONNAISE

MAYONNAISE, WHETHER OR NOT YOU LIKE IT ON A SANDWICH, CAN MAKE A GREAT DIPPING SAUCE OR SALAD DRESSING. THIS GARLIC-LEMON VERSION PACKS A FLAVOR PUNCH THAT'S GREAT WITH CRUNCHY CRUDITÉS, LIGHT GREEN SALADS, AND—MY PERSONAL FAVORITE—STEAMED ARTICHOKES. AND BECAUSE IT'S AIP-FRIENDLY, YOU CAN FEEL FREE TO DIP WITH ABANDON!

*ingredients*

⅓ cup (80 ml) avocado oil

⅓ cup (80 ml)
extra virgin olive oil

⅓ cup (80 ml)
palm shortening

1½ teaspoons (7.5 ml)
lemon juice

½ teaspoon garlic powder

Pinch of fine sea salt

*prep time*
5 minutes

*yield*
1 cup (240 ml)

## *directions*

1. Combine all the ingredients in a tall, narrow container and blend thoroughly with an immersion blender. Check the seasoning and adjust the salt to taste.

2. Store in an airtight container in the refrigerator. For a creamier consistency, remove from the refrigerator 20 minutes before serving.

*note*

GARLIC-LEMON MAYONNAISE
WILL KEEP IN THE REFRIGERATOR
FOR UP TO 7 DAYS.

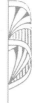

*The Autoimmune Protocol Made Simple Cookbook*

also shown

CREAMY CILANTRO
DRESSING (PAGE 44)
RANCH DRESSING
(PAGE 44)

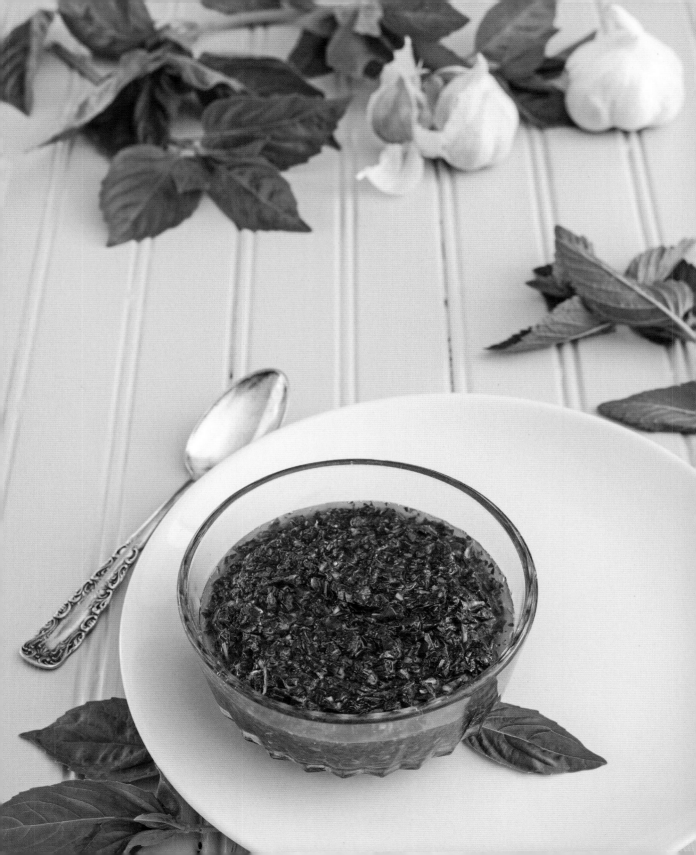

# CHIMICHURRI VERDE

THIS IS AN EXCELLENT SAUCE TO HAVE IN YOUR REPERTOIRE. IT MAKES A DELICIOUS MARINADE FOR BEEF, CHICKEN, LAMB, OR FISH, AND IT CAN ALSO BE USED AS A DIPPING OR FINISHING SAUCE. TRY IT ON TACOS AND AS A WAY TO LIVEN UP VEGGIES. BE ADVENTUROUS WITH THIS SAUCE—YOUR TASTE BUDS WILL THANK YOU!

## *directions*

1. Combine all the ingredients in a blender or food processor and blend on high for about 30 seconds, or until the sauce reaches your preferred consistency. You may have to stop once or twice to scrape down the sides of the blender or food processor with a spatula.

2. Transfer to an airtight container and refrigerate until needed.

### *ingredients*

4 cups (100 g) fresh basil

4 cups (60 g) fresh mint leaves

1 cup (240 ml) extra virgin olive oil

1½ tablespoons (22 ml) apple cider vinegar

4 cloves garlic, chopped

¼ teaspoon fine sea salt

### *prep time*
15 minutes

### *yield*
2 cups (480 ml)

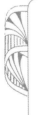

## *notes*

CHIMICHURRI VERDE WILL KEEP IN THE REFRIGERATOR FOR UP TO 1 WEEK.

TO AVOID OXIDATION, ALWAYS KEEP A THIN LAYER OF OLIVE OIL OVER THE TOP SURFACE.

## RANCH DRESSING

### ingredients
⅓ cup (80 ml) avocado oil

⅓ cup (80 ml) extra virgin olive oil

⅓ cup (80 ml) palm shortening

1½ teaspoons (7.5 ml) lemon juice

2 teaspoons (10 ml) coconut aminos

⅓ cup (20 g) minced parsley or (6 g) cilantro

Pinch of fine sea salt

### prep time
10 minutes

### yield
1 cup (240 ml)

---

JUST BECAUSE WE ARE ON A HEALING JOURNEY DOESN'T MEAN WE ARE SUDDENLY MORE VIRTUOUS. WE STILL WANT TO INDULGE NOW AND AGAIN. AND RANCH GOES WITH EVERYTHING, RIGHT? ENJOY THIS MOST VERSATILE OF DIPS WITHOUT DERAILING YOUR HEALTH. DIP AWAY!

### directions

1. Combine all the ingredients in a large bowl and beat with a hand mixer for about 30 seconds, until you obtain a smooth and creamy texture. Check the seasoning and adjust the salt to taste.

2. Store in an airtight container in the refrigerator. For a creamier consistency, remove from the refrigerator 20 minutes before serving.

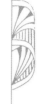

### note
RANCH DRESSING WILL KEEP IN THE REFRIGERATOR FOR UP TO 7 DAYS.

## CREAMY CILANTRO DRESSING

### ingredients
1 cup (240 ml) full-fat coconut milk

1 packed cup (16 g) chopped fresh cilantro

1 tablespoon (15 ml) lime juice

½ teaspoon fine sea salt, or more to taste

### prep time
5 minutes

### yield
1¼ cups (295 ml)

---

EATING FOR YOUR HEALTH DOESN'T MEAN YOU'RE CONDEMNED TO AUSTERITY. EVEN RAW VEGETABLES CAN BE TEMPTING IF YOU TREAT THEM RIGHT. A DECADENT SAUCE IS JUST THE TICKET TO LIFT YOUR FOOD FROM HO-HUM TO WOW! THIS DRESSING IS A FLAVOR BOOST FOR SO MANY THINGS, BUT ESPECIALLY VEGETABLES AND TACOS.

### directions

1. Combine all the ingredients in a high-speed blender and blend on high for about 30 seconds, until smooth. Taste and adjust the salt and lime juice to your liking.

2. Transfer the dressing to an airtight container and refrigerate until needed. Remove from the refrigerator 20 minutes before serving for a creamier consistency.

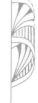

### note
CREAMY CILANTRO DRESSING WILL KEEP IN THE REFRIGERATOR FOR UP TO 5 DAYS.

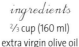

# SHALLOT VINAIGRETTE

A GOOD VINAIGRETTE WITH WELL-BALANCED ACIDITY AND SWEETNESS IS SOMETHING WORTH SEARCHING FOR. SEARCH NO FURTHER, MY FRIEND. THIS DRESSING IS THE ONE YOU'VE BEEN WAITING FOR. ELEGANT ENOUGH FOR COMPANY, BUT SIMPLE ENOUGH FOR EVERY DAY, THIS DRESSING IS DELICIOUS ON SALADS OR AS A LIGHT DIPPING SAUCE FOR CRUDITÉS.

## *ingredients*

2/3 cup (160 ml) extra virgin olive oil

1/3 cup (80 ml) apple cider vinegar

1 tablespoon (15 ml) honey

1/4 cup (40 g) minced shallots

1/4 cup (3 g) minced chives

1/4 teaspoon fine sea salt

### *prep time*
8 minutes

### *yield*
1 cup (240 ml)

## *directions*

1. Combine all the ingredients in a glass jar with a tight lid. Keep refrigerated until needed.

2. Remove from the refrigerator 10 minutes before serving to allow the olive oil to soften. Shake well before using.

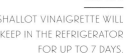

*notes*

SHALLOT VINAIGRETTE WILL KEEP IN THE REFRIGERATOR FOR UP TO 7 DAYS.

IF YOU DON'T HAVE SHALLOTS, USE RED ONION INSTEAD.

---

# CITRUS VINAIGRETTE

EVERYONE NEEDS A GOOD VINAIGRETTE IN THEIR REPERTOIRE— SOMETHING TO WHIP UP EASILY AND TRANSFORM ANY BLAND SALAD INTO SOMETHING CRAVE-WORTHY. LOOK NO FURTHER. THIS IS THE VINAIGRETTE YOU'VE BEEN WAITING FOR. WITH CITRUS TONES AND A HINT OF SALT, THIS DRESSING IS PERFECT FOR JUST ABOUT ANY SALAD YOU CAN DREAM UP.

## *ingredients*

1/2 cup (120 ml) extra virgin olive oil

1/3 cup (80 ml) freshly squeezed orange juice

2 tablespoons (30 ml) freshly squeezed lemon juice

Pinch of fine sea salt

### *prep time*
5 minutes

### *yield*
1 cup (240 ml)

## *directions*

1. Combine all the ingredients in a glass jar with a tight-fitting lid.

2. Keep refrigerated until needed. Remove from the refrigerator 10 minutes before serving to allow the olive oil to soften. Shake well before using.

*note*

CITRUS VINAIGRETTE WILL KEEP IN THE REFRIGERATOR FOR UP TO 7 DAYS.

# CHAPTER FIVE

# BREAKFASTS

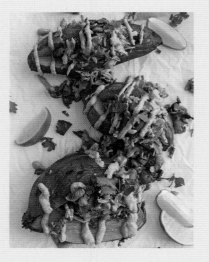

**FORGET ABOUT BAGELS,** cereal, and omelets. With AIP, your breakfast will begin to look a lot like dinner: vegetables, protein, and a good dose of healthy fats.

Breakfast is the most important meal of the day. But in my experience, people tend to skip it because it's just too much effort. Mornings are so hectic. Want an AIP-approved tip? The fastest way to get breakfast on the table is to simply warm up leftovers from the night before. Have a little more time to devote to your morning? Fuel up to the max with a meat and veggie skillet, or even better, a loaded sweet potato. Breakfast patties paired with veggies and healthy fats are always there for you when you are in a pinch. Cook them in advance, freeze them, and reheat as needed to save time.

If a savory breakfast doesn't tempt you, or for those lazy weekends, try my AIP-approved granola, pancakes, or oatmeal. You'll be surprised at how tasty and satisfying a healthy breakfast can be. And don't worry, die-hard coffee lovers will rejoice at my Caffeine-Free Iced Coffee and Pumpkin Spice Latte. And for those who like to drink their breakfast, a nutrient-packed smoothie will have you out the door in no time at all.

Whatever your fancy, try to focus on nutrient density for this crucial meal. Your body will thank you for it!

Welcome to AIP Breakfasts.

# FLUFFY PLANTAIN PANCAKES

YOU KNOW WHAT I LOVE? PANCAKES. FLUFFY, SLIGHTLY SWEET, DELICATE PANCAKES WITH MAPLE SYRUP. THESE PLANTAIN PANCAKES CAN FULFILL THAT CRAVING. THEY HAVE ALL THE QUALITIES OF A REGULAR PANCAKE, BUT WITH THE ADDED BONUS OF BEING COMPLETELY AIP COMPLIANT. PASS THE SYRUP, PLEASE!

## directions

1. Place the plantain, arrowroot flour, coconut flour, baking powder, and sea salt in a food processor. Set aside.

2. Heat the coconut milk in a small pan over medium-high heat for about 4 minutes, until hot but not boiling. Remove from the heat and sprinkle with the gelatin powder. Let it bloom for a couple of minutes, then whisk vigorously to dissolve the gelatin, ensuring there are no lumps.

3. Pour the coconut milk mixture over the dry ingredients and process for about 1 minute, until smooth and creamy. Use the batter immediately or cover and refrigerate for up to 12 hours in advance (prepare the night before for breakfast).

4. Heat 1 teaspoon coconut oil in a nonstick skillet over medium heat (increase the coconut oil if you are using a stainless steel skillet).

5. Drop 1 tablespoon (15 ml) of batter into the pan at a time. Spread the batter with a spoon so each little pancake is no larger than 2 inches (5 cm) wide and no thicker than 1/3 inch (8 mm). Cook for about 1½ minutes, until golden. Carefully flip the pancakes over with a spatula and cook for another minute, until golden.

6. Serve hot with your favorite topping.

## note

RIPE PLANTAINS SHOULD BE YELLOW WITH DARK SPOTS.

### ingredients

1 ripe plantain, peeled and chopped (see Note)

3 tablespoons (24 g) arrowroot flour

3 tablespoons (24 g) coconut flour

1/4 teaspoon baking powder

1/4 teaspoon fine sea salt

1/2 cup (120 ml) full-fat coconut milk

2 teaspoons (6 g) gelatin powder

Coconut oil, for cooking the pancakes

### prep time
15 minutes

### cook time
10 minutes

### yield
3 servings
(or 15 little pancakes)

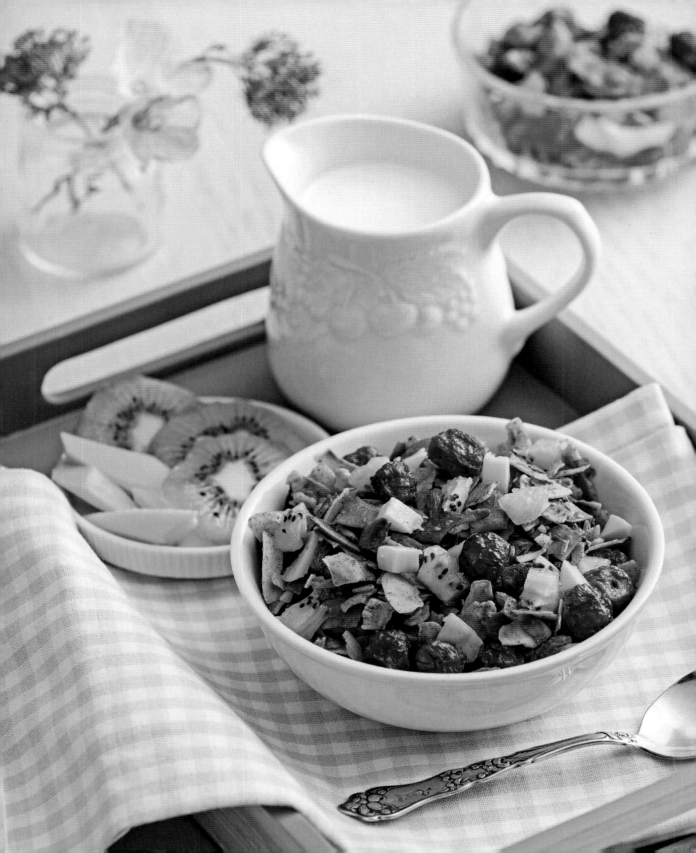

# GRAIN-FREE & NUT-FREE GRANOLA

BREAKFAST CAN BE TRICKY WHEN YOU ARE JUST STARTING AIP. THE ELIMINATION PERIOD IN PARTICULAR HAS YOU AVOIDING EGGS, WHICH FOR MANY PEOPLE ARE A BREAKFAST MAINSTAY. THIS GRAIN-FREE AND NUT-FREE GRANOLA WILL HELP YOU TRANSITION FROM YOUR OLD BREAKFAST STAPLES TO THE CLEANER OPTIONS THAT WILL BECOME YOUR NEW NORMAL.

## directions

1. Line a baking sheet with parchment paper and set aside.

2. Melt the coconut oil in a large skillet over medium heat. Add the coconut flakes, vanilla powder, and cinnamon. Mix well, ensuring the coconut flakes are well coated.

3. Cook, stirring frequently, for 8 to 10 minutes, until the coconut flakes are golden. Transfer to the prepared baking sheet. Let cool completely. Stir in the dehydrated cherries and raisins.

4. Store in an airtight container at room temperature.

5. Serve with coconut milk or coconut yogurt and fresh fruit.

## ingredients

2 tablespoons (30 ml) coconut oil

2 cups (170 g) unsweetened coconut flakes

½ teaspoon vanilla powder

1 teaspoon ground cinnamon

**ADD-INS:**

½ cup (80 g) dehydrated cherries

¼ cup (35 g) raisins

## prep time
5 minutes

## cook time
10 minutes

## yield
2¾ cups (652 g)

## note

HAVE FUN WITH THIS GRANOLA BY TRYING DIFFERENT ADD-INS, SUCH AS DRIED STRAWBERRIES, DRIED BLUEBERRIES, DRIED RASPBERRIES, CURRANTS, DRIED APPLES, OR DRIED BANANAS. BE SURE TO EAT THESE DRIED FRUITS ALONG WITH PARSIMONY SO AS NOT TO SPIKE BLOOD-SUGAR LEVELS.

# EXPRESS CAULIFLOWER "OATMEAL"

## ingredients

4 cups (470 g) raw
Cauliflower Rice
(page 106)

2 cups (470 ml) full-fat
coconut milk

**SUGGESTED TOPPINGS:**

Apple butter

Maple syrup

Honey

Fresh fruit

Shredded coconut

Grain-Free & Nut-Free
Granola (page 49)

### prep time
5 minutes

### cook time
20 minutes

### yield
4 (6-ounce, or 168 g)
servings

WHETHER YOU WANT A QUICK BREAKFAST OR JUST FEEL LIKE ADDING AN EXTRA DOSE OF VEGETABLES TO YOUR DIET, THIS SURPRISING CAULIFLOWER "OATMEAL" REALLY HITS THE SPOT. REMINISCENT OF TRADITIONAL OATMEAL, THIS ALLERGEN-FREE PORRIDGE WILL SATISFY YOUR TASTE BUDS WITH ITS WARM AND COMFORTING TEXTURE. PREPARE A LARGE BATCH IN ADVANCE AND REHEAT AS NEEDED, ADDING YOUR FAVORITE TOPPING AT THE LAST MINUTE.

## directions

1. Bring the cauliflower rice and coconut milk to a boil in a saucepan over high heat. Reduce the heat to medium and cook, uncovered, for about 20 minutes, until the cauliflower is tender.

2. Serve immediately with your favorite topping or refrigerate for later use.

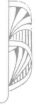

## note
EXPRESS CAULIFLOWER "OATMEAL" WILL KEEP FOR UP TO 5 DAYS, STORED IN AN AIRTIGHT CONTAINER IN THE REFRIGERATOR.

*The Autoimmune Protocol Made Simple Cookbook*

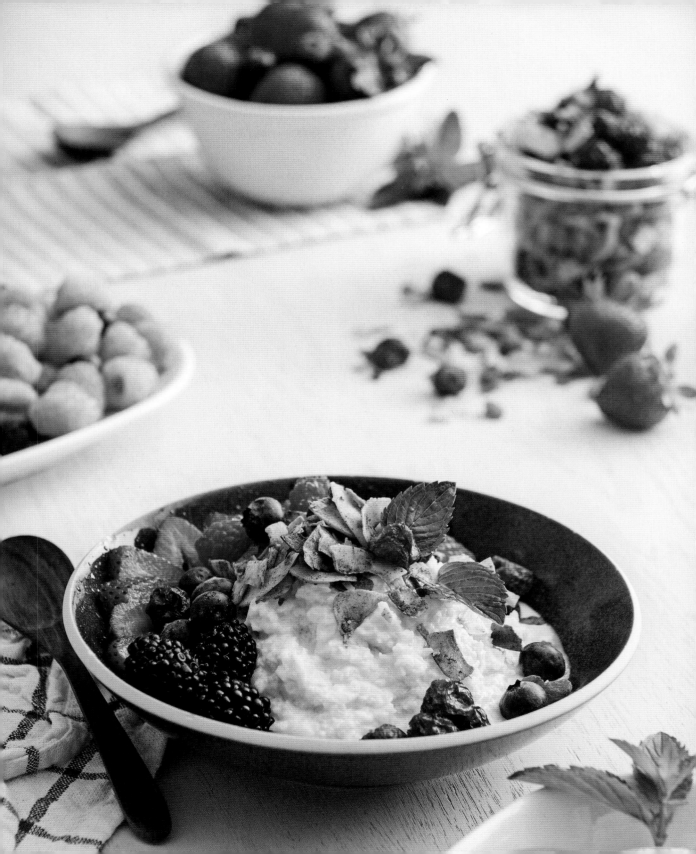

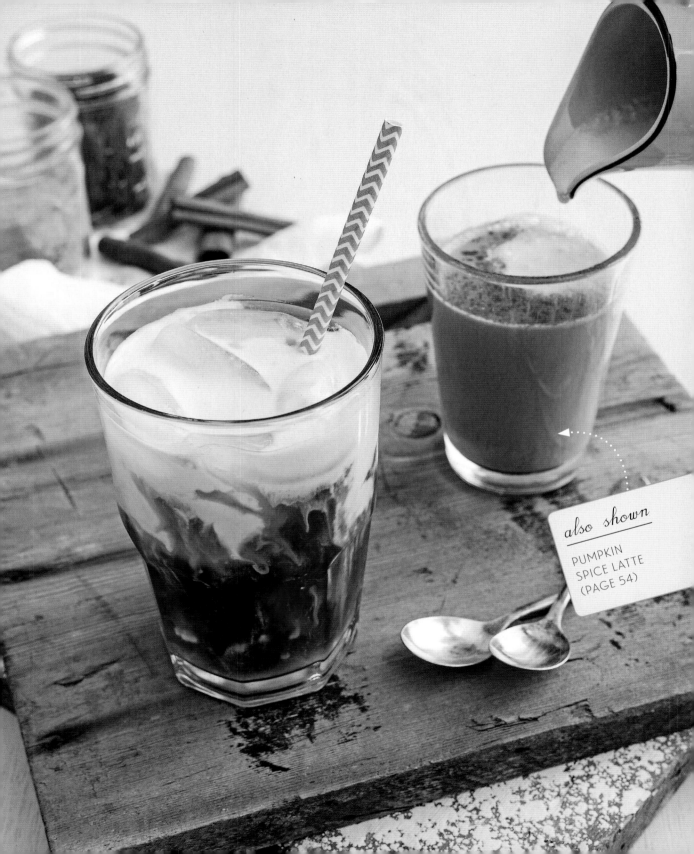

*also shown*

PUMPKIN
SPICE LATTE
(PAGE 54)

# CAFFEINE-FREE ICED COFFEE

COFFEE IS ONE OF THE HARDEST THINGS TO GIVE UP DURING THE ELIMINATION PHASE OF THE AUTOIMMUNE PROTOCOL. PART OF WHAT MAKES IT SO HARD IS THE RITUAL: THE SMELL OF THE BEANS, HOLDING A MUG OF SOMETHING YOU KNOW IS GOING TO MAKE YOU FEEL GOOD. IT'S HARD TO LET GO OF ALL THAT. NOW YOU DON'T HAVE TO. YOU CAN ENJOY THE SAME FEELING WITH THIS CAFFEINE-FREE COFFEE.

## directions

1. Place the dandelion root and chicory root in a French press. Pour the boiling water into the press and brew for about 5 minutes, until dark.

2. Fill a tall glass with ice cubes. Pour the coffee over the ice, then stir in a generous portion of the Dairy-Free Vanilla-Maple Creamer.

### ingredients

½ tablespoon (4 g) ground or granulated dandelion root

1 teaspoon roasted chicory root

1¼ cups (300 ml) boiling water

Ice to taste

Dairy-Free Vanilla-Maple Creamer (page 35) to taste

### prep time
5 minutes

### yield
1 serving

## notes

DANDELION ROOT OFTEN COMES IN SMALL BITS AND PIECES. I LIKE TO GRIND IT IN A COFFEE GRINDER TO OBTAIN A MORE USABLE POWDER.

IF YOU DON'T HAVE A FRENCH PRESS, USE A LOOSE-LEAF TEA BAG TO BREW YOUR COFFEE.

NOT IN THE MOOD FOR A COLD DRINK? SKIP THE ICE AND ENJOY THIS CAFFEINE-FREE COFFEE HOT—WITH OR WITHOUT CREAMER!

# PUMPKIN SPICE LATTE

NOTHING SAYS FALL BETTER THAN A WARM, COMFORTING SPICED LATTE. THIS CAFFEINE-FREE AND DAIRY-FREE VERSION IS EASY TO MAKE ON THE STOVETOP. WHY NOT MAKE A BIG BATCH AND THEN REHEAT A CUP WHEN YOU NEED A LITTLE SOMETHING WARM? WITH REAL PUMPKIN PUREE, VANILLA-MAPLE CREAMER, CINNAMON, AND CLOVES, THIS YUMMY DRINK HITS ALL THE RIGHT SPOTS FOR A GUILT-FREE, INDULGENT MOMENT.

## *ingredients*

½ tablespoon (4 g) ground or granulated dandelion root

1 teaspoon roasted chicory root

1¼ cups (300 ml) boiling water

¼ cup (60 ml) Dairy-Free Vanilla-Maple Creamer (page 35)

3 tablespoons (50 g) pumpkin puree

2 teaspoons (10 ml) maple syrup

Pinch of ground cinnamon, plus more for serving

Pinch of ground cloves

Coconut Whipped Cream (page 155), for serving

*prep time*
5 minutes

*yield*
1 serving

## *directions*

1. Place the dandelion root and chicory root in a French press. Pour the boiling water into the press and let brew for about 5 minutes, until dark.

2. Transfer the coffee to a small pan. Add the Dairy-Free Vanilla-Maple Creamer, pumpkin puree, maple syrup, cinnamon, and ground cloves. Heat the mixture over low heat, stirring, for a few minutes.

3. Serve hot with a scoop of Coconut Whipped Cream and a dash of cinnamon.

## *notes*

INSTEAD OF BREWING DANDELION AND CHICORY ROOTS IN A FRENCH PRESS, YOU CAN ALTERNATIVELY USE A LOOSE-LEAF TEA BAG IN A GLASS CONTAINER.

DANDELION ROOT OFTEN COMES IN GRANULATED FORM. I GRIND MINE IN A SMALL COFFEE GRINDER AND STORE IT IN AN AIRTIGHT GLASS CONTAINER.

FREEZE THE EXTRA CANNED PUMPKIN PUREE IN ICE CUBE TRAYS AND KEEP FOR FUTURE USE.

*The Autoimmune Protocol Made Simple Cookbook*

# HIDDEN VEGGIES SMOOTHIE

AIP ASKS THAT WE CONSUME A LOT OF VEGGIES, AND I AM ALWAYS LOOKING FOR CREATIVE WAYS TO SNEAK MORE OF THEM INTO MY DIET. THIS SMOOTHIE IS A GREAT OPTION IF YOU ARE IN A HURRY OR ARE TIRING OF MORE TRADITIONAL VEGETABLE PREPARATIONS. YOU'LL NEVER EVEN KNOW THEY'RE IN THERE! FOR A BOOST OF PROTEIN, ADD COLLAGEN PEPTIDES. CRAVING SOME CRUNCH? ADD SOME GRAIN-FREE & NUT-FREE GRANOLA (PAGE 49).

## directions

1. Combine all the ingredients in a blender and blend until smooth.

2. Serve immediately as is or with your favorite topping.

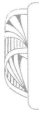

### note

FOR A CREAMIER SMOOTHIE, REPLACE THE COCONUT WATER WITH COCONUT MILK.

### ingredients

1 cup (240 ml) coconut water

2 cups (70 g) chopped kale

1 banana, peeled

1 cup (150 g) frozen blueberries

¼ avocado, peeled

5 mint leaves

1 tablespoon (11 g) collagen peptides (optional)

### prep time
5 minutes

### yield
1 (20-ounce, or 560 g) serving

# CARROT CAKE SMOOTHIE

MORNINGS CAN BE HECTIC WITH KIDS, LUNCHES, WORK, AND ALL THE REST OF IT. IT SEEMS LIKE WE'RE ALWAYS IN A HURRY, BUT SOMETIMES WE CRAVE A LITTLE SOMETHING SPECIAL. THERE AREN'T TOO MANY BREAKFAST TREATS SANCTIONED BY THE AUTOIMMUNE PROTOCOL, BUT THIS CARROT CAKE SMOOTHIE SURE FITS THE BILL. IT'S SUPER HEALTHY, WITH A SERVING OF CARROTS AND AVOCADO, AND SUPER DELICIOUS TO BOOT.

## *ingredients*

1 cup (240 ml) coconut water

½ small banana

½ cup (65 g) chopped carrots

½ cup (125 g) frozen peaches

¼ avocado, peeled

Pinch of ground cinnamon

Pinch of ground cloves

Pinch of dried ground ginger

1 tablespoon (11 g) collagen peptides (optional)

*prep time*
5 minutes

*yield*
1 (20-ounce, or 560 g) serving

## *directions*

1. Combine all the ingredients in a blender and blend until smooth.

2. Serve immediately as is or with your favorite topping.

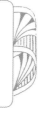

*note*

FOR A CREAMIER SMOOTHIE, REPLACE THE COCONUT WATER WITH COCONUT MILK.

*The Autoimmune Protocol Made Simple Cookbook*

# PORK-VEGGIE BREAKFAST SKILLET

BREAKFAST SKILLETS ARE MY FAVORITE. THEY ARE VERSATILE, SATISFYING, AND OH SO FORGIVING. YOUR CHOPPING DOESN'T HAVE TO BE PERFECT; YOUR PANS DON'T HAVE TO BE ANY SPECIFIC SIZE. ALL YOU HAVE TO DO IS TOSS EVERYTHING TOGETHER, AND IT WILL BE JUST RIGHT. THIS VEGGIE-FORWARD VERSION IS JUST THE THING TO GET YOU GOING IN THE MORNING. TRY SWAPPING OUT THE SQUASH FOR SWEET POTATOES OR CARROTS.

## directions

1. Heat 1 tablespoon (15 ml) of the olive oil in a large skillet over medium heat. Add the ground pork, ¾ teaspoon of the sea salt, and the garlic powder and cook, stirring frequently, for about 5 minutes or until the meat is cooked through and no longer pink. Transfer to a plate with a slotted spoon. Cover and keep warm in the oven at 200°F (95°C).

2. Add the remaining 1 tablespoon (15 ml) olive oil to the skillet. Add the onion and cook, stirring frequently, for 5 minutes.

3. Add the zucchini and continue to cook, covered, for 10 minutes. Add the butternut squash, water, and remaining ½ teaspoon sea salt. Mix well and continue to cook, covered, for about 5 minutes, or until tender.

4. Add the cooked meat back to the skillet, toss to combine, and serve immediately with a generous garnish of cilantro.

### ingredients

2 tablespoons (30 ml) extra virgin olive oil, divided

1 pound (450 g) ground pork

1¼ teaspoons (8 g) fine sea salt, divided

½ teaspoon garlic powder

1½ cups (240 g) finely chopped yellow onion

4 cups (500 g) chopped zucchini

2 cups (280 g) shredded butternut squash (see Note)

⅓ cup (80 ml) water

Chopped fresh cilantro, for garnish

### prep time
15 minutes

### cook time
25 minutes

### yield
4 or 5 servings

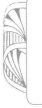

## note

TO QUICKLY SHRED BUTTERNUT SQUASH, USE A FOOD PROCESSOR WITH A SHREDDING DISK.

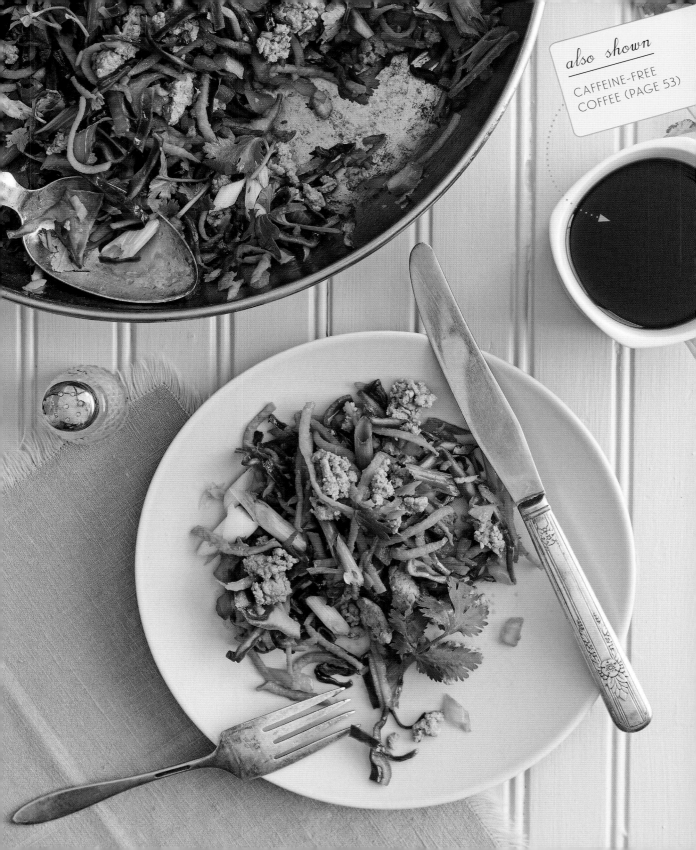

*also shown*

CAFFEINE-FREE
COFFEE (PAGE 53)

# TURKEY-VEGGIE BREAKFAST SKILLET

WHO NEEDS EGGS? THIS HEARTY, SAVORY BREAKFAST WILL KEEP YOU GOING STRONG UNTIL LUNCH. YOU CAN DRAMATICALLY REDUCE THE TIME YOUR MORNING ROUTINE TAKES BY PREPPING YOUR INGREDIENTS IN ADVANCE AND STORING THEM IN RESEALABLE PLASTIC BAGS OR GLASS CONTAINERS IN YOUR REFRIGERATOR. JUST GRAB THE BAGS AND EMPTY THEM INTO A SKILLET, AND YOUR BREAKFAST WILL BE READY IN MINUTES!

## directions

1. Heat 1½ tablespoons (23 ml) of the olive oil in a large skillet over medium heat. Add the ground turkey and ¾ teaspoon of the sea salt. Cook, stirring frequently, for about 5 minutes, until the meat is cooked through and no longer pink. Transfer to a plate with a slotted spoon. Cover and keep warm in the oven at 200°F (95°C).

2. Add the remaining 1½ tablespoons (22 ml) olive oil to the skillet. Add the onion and cook, stirring regularly, for 5 minutes.

3. Add the red cabbage and coconut aminos. Cover and cook for 10 minutes.

4. Add the sweet potato, water, and remaining ½ teaspoon sea salt. Mix well and continue to cook, covered, for about 5 minutes, or until tender.

5. Add the cooked meat back to the skillet, toss to combine, and serve immediately with a generous garnish of chopped cilantro and scallions.

## ingredients

3 tablespoons (45 ml) extra virgin olive oil, divided

1 pound (450 g) ground turkey

1¼ teaspoons (8 g) fine sea salt, divided

1½ cups (240 g) finely chopped yellow onion

3 cups (270 g) sliced red cabbage

2 tablespoons (30 ml) coconut aminos

2 cups (270 g) shredded raw sweet potato (see Note)

⅓ cup (80 ml) water

Chopped fresh cilantro, for garnish

Chopped scallions, for garnish

prep time
15 minutes

cook time
25 minutes

yield
4 or 5 servings

## note

TO QUICKLY SHRED SWEET POTATOES, USE A FOOD PROCESSOR WITH A SHREDDING DISK.

# LOADED SWEET POTATOES

THE BEST WAY TO SAVE TIME WITH THIS DISH IS TO PRECOOK THE SWEET POTATOES AND HAVE THE OTHER INGREDIENTS READY IN THE REFRIGERATOR. THAT WAY, YOU JUST HAVE TO WARM UP EVERYTHING AT THE LAST MINUTE. ENJOY THIS NUTRITIOUS AND FILLING MEAL AS BREAKFAST, LUNCH, OR DINNER. HOWEVER YOU DO IT, YOU'LL BE FULL AND SATISFIED.

## *ingredients*

4 medium-size (6 to 8 ounces, or 170 to 225 g) sweet potatoes

4 slices bacon (about 5 ounces, or 140 g), cut into ¼-inch (6 mm) strips

5 ounces (140 g) mushrooms, thinly sliced

½ cup (60 g) thinly sliced red onion

1⅓ cups (215 g) Versatile Pulled Pork Carnitas (page 126)

Fine sea salt to taste

Spicy Guacamole (page 39) to taste

Chopped fresh Italian parsley, for garnish

Creamy Cilantro Dressing (page 44) to taste

*prep time*
10 minutes

*cook time*
60 to 70 minutes

*yield*
4 servings

## *directions*

1. Place the oven rack in the middle position and preheat the oven to 400°F (200°C).

2. Pierce the sweet potatoes a few times with a fork and wrap them loosely in aluminum foil. Place them on a baking sheet and bake for 60 to 70 minutes, until tender. Allow to cool before discarding the aluminum foil.

3. While the sweet potatoes are in the oven, cook the bacon in a skillet over medium heat for 8 to 10 minutes, until crisp. Transfer the bacon to a paper towel–lined plate with a slotted spoon, reserving the bacon fat in the pan.

4. Add the mushrooms and onions to the skillet with the reserved bacon fat. Cover and cook over medium heat, stirring frequently, for about 10 minutes, until golden and tender. Add the bacon back to the skillet and mix well.

5. Reheat the Versatile Pulled Pork Carnitas using your preferred method.

6. To load the sweet potatoes: Cut each potato in half lengthwise (don't cut all the way through; leave a ¼-inch [6 mm] space uncut). Season with a dash of sea salt, then top with the Versatile Pulled Pork Carnitas, Spicy Guacamole, bacon mixture, parsley, and a drizzle of Creamy Cilantro Dressing. Serve hot.

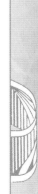

### note

IF YOU DECIDE TO PREPARE
THESE SWEET POTATOES
IN ADVANCE, WRAP
THEM INDIVIDUALLY IN
ALUMINUM FOIL, ADDING
THE GUACAMOLE, FRESH
PARSLEY, AND CILANTRO
DRESSING AT THE LAST
MINUTE AFTER YOU HAVE
REHEATED THE SWEET
POTATO.

# CHICKEN-APPLE PATTIES

SAUSAGE PATTIES CAN STILL BE A GO-TO FAVORITE FOR BREAKFAST ON THE AIP. ADDED BONUS: YOU CAN AVOID NON-AIP HIDDEN INGREDIENTS WITH THIS HOMEMADE VERSION. LIGHT AND BARELY SWEET (THANKS TO THE APPLES), THIS IS THE PERFECT PATTY TO START YOUR DAY OFF ON THE RIGHT FOOT. ADD VEGETABLES, OF COURSE, FOR A COMPLETE AND WHOLESOME MEAL. THESE PATTIES FREEZE WELL, SO THEY ARE PERFECT FOR BATCH COOKING.

### *ingredients*

1 pound (450 g) ground chicken

½ Granny Smith apple, finely diced

1 teaspoon dried sage

¾ teaspoon sea salt

½ teaspoon dried onion flakes

### *prep time*
10 minutes

### *cook time*
20 minutes

### *yield*
6 patties

## *directions*

1. Place the oven rack in the top third of the oven, and preheat the oven to 350°F (175°C). Grease a baking sheet with olive oil and set aside.

2. Combine all the ingredients in a bowl and mix thoroughly using a lightly oiled wooden spatula.

3. Using a ⅓-cup (80 g) measure, divide the meat mixture into 6 portions and place them directly onto the baking sheet. Lightly oil your fingers and flatten the meat into patties. This way, you won't have too much meat sticking to your fingers and hands. You should have enough for about 6 patties.

4. Bake for 20 minutes, or until the patties have reached an internal temperature of 165°F (74°C), turning the patties over halfway through the cooking time.

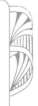

### *notes*

IF YOU DON'T HAVE GROUND CHICKEN ON HAND, SWAP FOR GROUND PORK OR TURKEY.

SERVE WITH BAKED SPAGHETTI SQUASH (PAGE 101), SPEEDY CAULIFLOWER RICE (PAGE 106), OR CREAMY MASHED BROCCOLI (PAGE 107).

# MAPLE-BACON PATTIES

DON'T MAKE THE MISTAKE OF RESERVING THESE PATTIES ONLY
FOR BREAKFAST. EVEN THOUGH THEY CONTAIN A HINT OF MAPLE
SYRUP, THESE PORK PATTIES WILL COME IN HANDY AT EVERY MEAL,
ESPECIALLY IF YOU ARE SHORT ON TIME. AND DID I MENTION THE
BACON? HIGHLY PORTABLE, THEY ALSO MAKE GREAT LUNCH BOX
STUFFERS AND PICNIC FOOD. MAKE A DOUBLE BATCH AND FREEZE
HALF BEFORE COOKING. JUST BE SURE TO SEPARATE THE PATTIES
YOU ARE FREEZING WITH PIECES OF PARCHMENT PAPER.

## *directions*

1. Place the oven rack in the top third of the oven, and preheat the oven
   to 350°F (175°C). Grease a baking sheet with olive oil and set it aside.

2. Combine all the ingredients in a large bowl and mix thoroughly with
   your hands.

3. Divide the meat mixture into 6 portions, form them into patties, and
   arrange them on the baking sheet.

4. Bake for 20 minutes or until the patties have reached an internal
   temperature of 160°F (71°C), turning the patties over halfway through
   the cooking time.

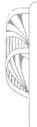

## *notes*

IF YOU DON'T HAVE GROUND PORK ON HAND,
SWAP FOR GROUND CHICKEN OR BEEF.

WHEN FREEZING, SEPARATE PATTIES WITH
LAYERS OF PARCHMENT PAPER.

## *ingredients*

1 pound (450 g) ground pork

2½ ounces (70 g)
bacon, thinly sliced

1 tablespoon (15 ml)
maple syrup

¾ teaspoon fine sea salt

½ teaspoon dried marjoram

## *prep time*
10 minutes

## *cook time*
20 minutes

## *yield*
6 patties

# CHAPTER SIX

# SMALL BITES

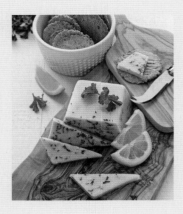

**I AM OFTEN HUNGRY** right around 3 o'clock in the afternoon. I want—no, I *need*—a snack, but I don't want to throw any old thing into my mouth. I want it to be healthy, nourishing, and satisfying. The small bites in this chapter fit that bill. They will help keep your energy up without the crash of sugary, carbohydrate-rich snacks favored by the Standard American Diet.

This chapter is full of wonderful, simple, healthy recipes that will take you from snack time to dinnertime. From chicken poppers and tasty tostones to AIP nachos and sweet potato sliders, this chapter has something for even the pickiest eater out there. I even have hummus and pickles for you. Skip the store-bought versions and make your own! They will come in handy for those yummy Rainbow Veggie Wraps on page 74.

What's that? You miss cheese? I've got you covered. My zucchini cheese will fool almost anyone and can even be shredded! And my Cocktail Cheese Bites are just the thing to pop into your mouth before dinner. If you're adventurous, try my Beginner's Liver Pâté for a tasty introduction to liver. A small bite is the perfect way to jump into something new, so give it a try.

These recipes will also do nicely for a party. Consider serving any of them the next time you entertain. No one will notice they are AIP approved, and you will be able to relax, socialize, and enjoy some fun, delicious appetizers without putting your healing at risk.

Welcome to AIP Small Bites.

# CHICKEN-VEGGIE POPPERS

DEFINITELY A CROWD-PLEASER, THESE LITTLE NUGGETS ARE PACKED
WITH GOOD-FOR-YOU VEGGIES AND PROTEIN. DELICIOUS ON
THEIR OWN WITH A LITTLE SALT OR DRESSED UP WITH A DIPPING
SAUCE SUCH AS RANCH DRESSING (PAGE 44), GARLIC-LEMON
MAYONNAISE (PAGE 40), SPICY GUACAMOLE (PAGE 39), OR
CHIMICHURRI VERDE (PAGE 43), THESE POPPERS ARE A PERFECT
SNACK. THEY'RE EVEN BETTER AS AN APPETIZER FOR A PARTY, BUT
MAKE SURE YOU GET YOUR SHARE! THESE GUYS WILL DISAPPEAR
FROM THE PLATE FASTER THAN YOU CAN BLINK.

## *directions*

1. Place the oven rack in the top third of the oven and preheat it to 400°F
   (200°C). Line 2 baking sheets with parchment paper and set aside.

2. Mix all the ingredients thoroughly in a large bowl with a spoon. Scoop
   out small portions with a tablespoon and form little patties about ⅓ inch
   (8 mm) thick and 2 inches (5 cm) wide with your hands. Arrange them on
   the baking sheets.

3. Bake, flipping halfway through, for about 20 minutes, or until golden
   and crispy.

4. Enjoy warm or cold with a dipping sauce or without.

## *ingredients*

12 ounces (340 g)
ground chicken

2 cups (220 g)
raw shredded carrots

1 cup (100 g)
raw cauliflower rice

⅓ cup (40 g)
arrowroot flour

1 tablespoon (1.5 g)
dried coriander leaves

1½ tablespoons (22 ml)
coconut aminos

¾ teaspoon fine sea salt

1 teaspoon garlic powder

1 teaspoon onion powder

## *prep time*
15 minutes

## *cook time*
20 minutes

## *yield*
30 poppers

## *note*

MAKE THE PATTIES A BIT BIGGER
AND USE THEM TO TOP A SALAD
FOR A DELICIOUS MAIN DISH.

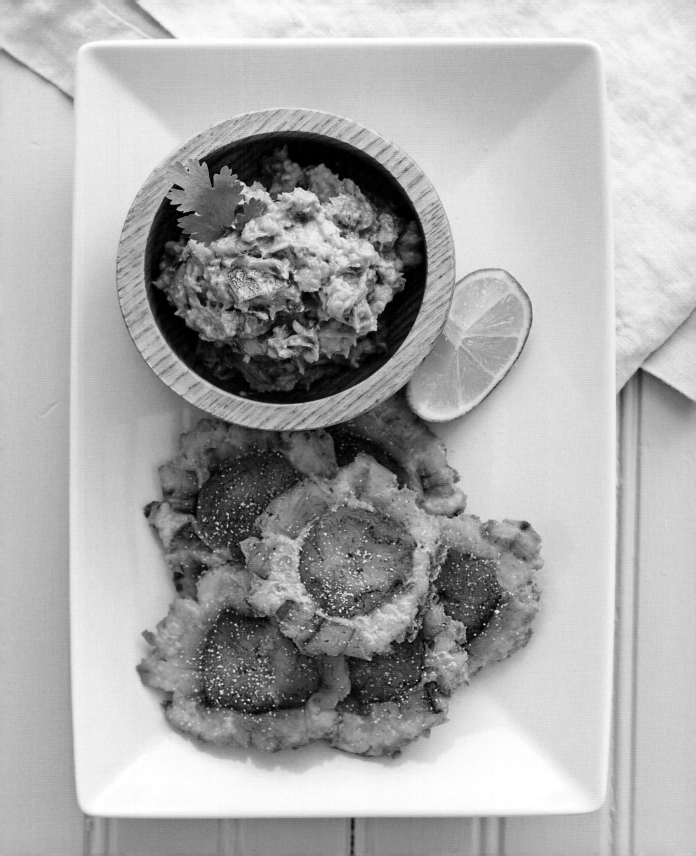

# LIME–SEA SALT TOSTONES

TOSTONES ARE TWICE-FRIED PLANTAIN CHIPS. THESE CHIPS ARE SALTY, CRISPY, CRUNCHY LITTLE BITS OF JOY. HONESTLY, THEY WILL MAKE YOU HAPPY. GREEN PLANTAINS WITH A FEW BLACK SPOTS WORK BEST FOR THIS RECIPE. IF YOU DECIDE TO DOUBLE IT, YOU MAY HAVE TO WORK IN SEVERAL BATCHES SO AS NOT TO OVERCROWD THE PAN.

## directions

1. Peel the plantain with a vegetable peeler. Slice into twelve 1-inch (2.5 cm)-thick pieces.

2. Heat the coconut oil in a large nonstick pan over medium heat. Carefully place pieces of plantain into the hot oil so they don't touch each other. Fry until golden, about 3 minutes on each side.

3. Transfer the plantains to a paper towel–lined plate with a slotted spoon. One by one, flatten each piece to ¼ inch (6 mm) thick between 2 sheets of parchment paper.

4. Return the flattened plantain slices to the hot oil and fry for another 1 to 2 minutes on each side. Remove from the pan with a slotted spoon. Drain the excess oil on paper towels and transfer to a serving dish.

5. Season to taste with garlic powder and sea salt. Drizzle with lime juice. Serve hot or cold.

### ingredients
1 green plantain
¼ cup (60 ml) coconut oil
Garlic powder to taste
Fine sea salt to taste
Lime juice to taste

### prep time
5 minutes

### cook time
10 minutes

### yield
12 pieces

## notes

SERVE AS A SIDE DISH OR AS AN APPETIZER WITH SPICY GUACAMOLE (PAGE 39).

THIS RECIPE WORKS BEST IN A NONSTICK SKILLET. IF YOU ARE USING A STAINLESS STEEL OR CAST-IRON SKILLET, MAKE SURE YOU HAVE A GOOD AMOUNT OF FAT AT ALL TIMES AND CLEAN THE PAN BETWEEN BATCHES.

# AIP NACHOS

WHO DOESN'T LOVE NACHOS?! PERFECT FOR MOVIE NIGHTS AND THOSE HOT SUMMER DAYS WHEN YOU DON'T WANT ANYTHING HEAVY, THESE NACHOS ARE CRUNCHY, SAVORY, AND JUST AS DELICIOUS AS YOU REMEMBER. AND YOU THOUGHT STARTING AIP MEANT NO MORE NACHOS. SILLY YOU! THESE 100 PERCENT AIP-COMPLIANT NACHOS WILL MAKE YOU BELIEVE ANYTHING IS POSSIBLE WITH A LITTLE EFFORT—EVEN GOOD HEALTH.

## *ingredients*

1 tablespoon (15 m) extra virgin olive oil

1 pound (450 g) ground meat of choice

¾ teaspoon fine sea salt

1 teaspoon turmeric powder

½ teaspoon garlic powder

½ teaspoon onion powder

4 cups (280 g) thinly sliced romaine lettuce

⅓ cup (70 g) minced red onion

¾ cup (100 g) sliced kalamata olives

Spicy Guacamole (page 39)

Minced fresh cilantro, for garnish

Lime–Sea Salt Tostones (page 67)

## *directions*

1. Heat the olive oil in a skillet over medium heat. Add the ground meat, sea salt, turmeric powder, garlic powder, and onion powder. Cook, stirring frequently and breaking the meat into small pieces, for about 8 minutes, until the meat is no longer pink.

2. To assemble the nachos: Layer the ingredients evenly on 4 dinner plates in the following order: lettuce, meat, red onion, olives, and Spicy Guacamole. Sprinkle with cilantro. Serve with tostones on the side for scooping up the good stuff, or you can even include them as a layer for easy scooping.

## *prep time*
20 minutes

## *cook time*
8 minutes

## *yield*
4 servings

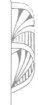

## *note*

TOSTONES MAY BE REPLACED WITH AIP-COMPLIANT SWEET POTATO CHIPS.

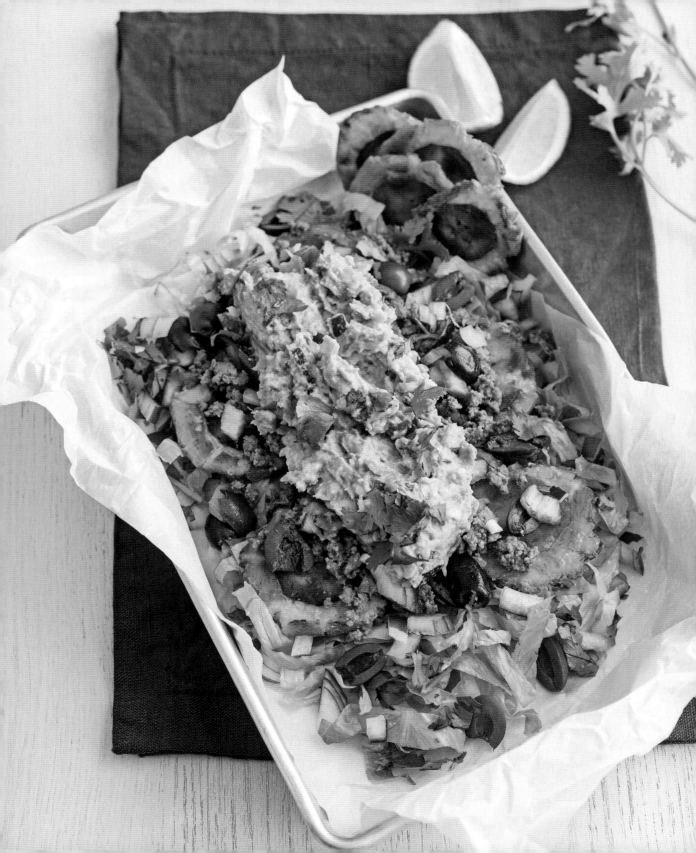

# CHEESY BACON SWEET POTATO SLIDERS

SURPRISE YOUR FRIENDS AT YOUR NEXT PARTY WITH THESE FUN LITTLE SLIDERS. NO ONE WILL BELIEVE YOU ARE ALLOWED TO EAT SUCH SINFULLY DELICIOUS TREATS ON YOUR "DIET." RICH WITH FLAVOR AND EVER-SO-FUN TO EAT, THIS IS FINGER FOOD AT ITS BEST. BE HONEST, DID YOU THINK ADOPTING AIP WOULD BE THIS MUCH FUN?

## *ingredients*

1 tablespoon (15 ml) coconut oil

1 sweet potato (about 12 ounces, or 340 g), cut into 10 ¼-inch (6 mm) slices

Fine sea salt to taste

4 ounces (115 g) broccoli florets

3 slices bacon (about 5 ounces, or 140 g), cut into ¼-inch (6 mm) strips

"Cheesy" Sauce (page 39) to taste

Minced chives, for garnish

*prep time*
10 minutes

*cook time*
30 minutes

*yield*
10 sliders

## *directions*

1. Place the oven rack in the top third of the oven and preheat it to 400°F (200°C). Grease the bottom of a rimmed roasting pan with the coconut oil.

2. Arrange the sweet potato slices flat on the roasting pan so they don't overlap and season them with sea salt. Roast, flipping halfway through, for about 30 minutes, or until tender and golden.

3. Meanwhile, steam the broccoli florets (see Note) for about 10 minutes, until tender. Drain and keep warm.

4. Cook the bacon in a skillet for 8 to 10 minutes, until golden. Transfer to a paper towel–lined plate with a slotted spoon. Warm up the "Cheesy" Sauce.

5. To assemble: Place a piece of broccoli on top of each sweet potato slice, followed by a spoonful of "Cheesy" Sauce, bacon, chives, and a pinch of sea salt.

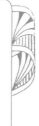

## *note*

TO STEAM BROCCOLI FLORETS: TRIM THE BROCCOLI, REMOVE THE TOUGH OUTER SKIN FROM THE STALKS, AND CHOP. PLACE A VEGETABLE STEAMER IN A POT, ADD 1 TO 2 INCHES (2.5 TO 5 CM) OF WATER, AND BRING TO A BOIL. ADD THE BROCCOLI, COVER, AND STEAM FOR ABOUT 10 MINUTES, UNTIL TENDER.

# GARLIC REFRIGERATOR PICKLES

AIP-COMPLIANT PICKLES ARE DIFFICULT TO FIND IN STORES BECAUSE THEY OFTEN CONTAIN SPICES THAT HAVE BEEN REMOVED FROM YOUR DIET DURING THE ELIMINATION PHASE OF THE AUTOIMMUNE PROTOCOL. THE GOOD NEWS IS, THEY ARE EASY TO MAKE. FEEL FREE TO EXPERIMENT WITH ANY KIND OF FRESH HERBS YOU HAVE ON HAND; YOU REALLY CAN'T GO WRONG. P.S. LACTOFERMENTED VEGETABLES ARE A GOOD SOURCE OF NATURAL PROBIOTICS.

## directions

1. To make the brine: Bring the water and apple cider vinegar to a boil in a saucepan over high heat and add the sea salt. Stir until the salt dissolves. Remove from the heat and let cool for a few minutes.

2. To make the vegetables: Divide the cucumbers, garlic, and fresh herbs between 2 pint-size (450 ml) jars so they are packed full. Pour the brine over the vegetables to cover completely. Let cool, then seal the jars with the lids.

3. Refrigerate for at least 3 days before digging in.

## note

GARLIC REFRIGERATOR PICKLES WILL KEEP FOR UP TO 2 WEEKS IN THE REFRIGERATOR.

## ingredients

**FOR THE BRINE:**

1½ cups (350 ml) water

1 cup (240 ml) apple cider vinegar

1 tablespoon (18 g) fine sea salt

**FOR THE VEGETABLES:**

1 pound (450 g) pickling cucumbers, quartered lengthwise or thinly sliced

6 cloves garlic, thinly sliced

6 large sprigs fresh dill

6 large sprigs fresh tarragon

## prep time
10 minutes

## cook time
5 minutes

## yield
2 pint-size (450 ml) jars

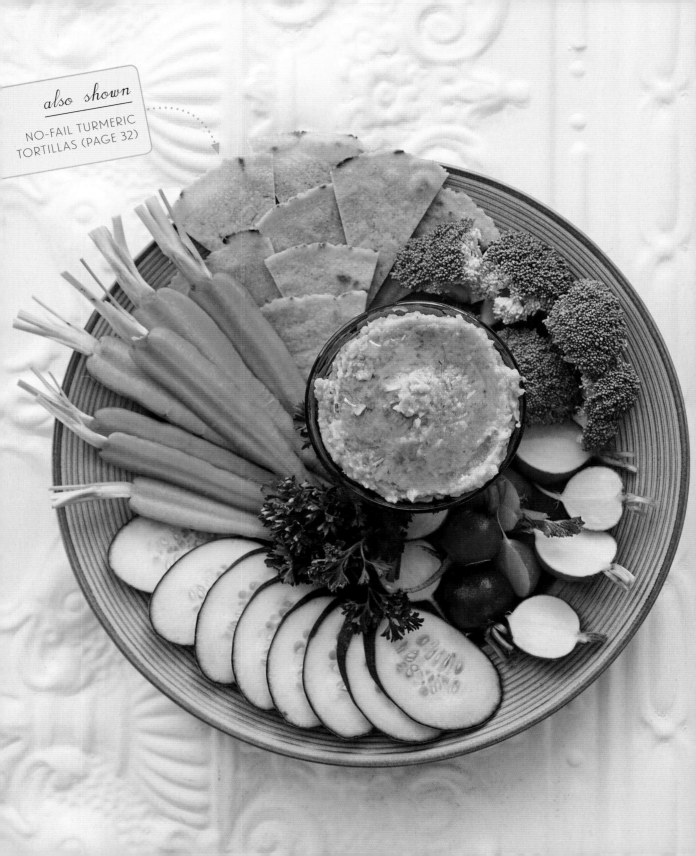

*also shown*

NO-FAIL TURMERIC
TORTILLAS (PAGE 32)

# ROASTED FENNEL HUMMUS

TRADITIONALLY, HUMMUS IS MADE WITH BEANS, A NO-NO ON AIP. THIS DELICIOUS VEGETABLE-BASED HUMMUS REMOVES THE BEANS AND CREATES AN ENTIRELY DIFFERENT (AND ENTIRELY AIP-SAFE!) DIP THAT CAN BE ENJOYED WITH CRUDITÉS, AS A SPREAD FOR SANDWICHES, OR ON A SPOON STRAIGHT OUT OF THE BOWL. GO AHEAD AND INDULGE A LITTLE—IT'S GOOD FOR YOU!

## directions

1. Place the rack in the middle position of the oven and preheat it to 350°F (175°C). Grease the bottom of a rimmed roasting pan with olive oil.

2. Arrange the fennel, sweet potato, and garlic in the pan in a single layer. Bake, stirring a couple of times partway through, for about 40 minutes, until the vegetables are tender.

3. Allow the vegetables to cool, then transfer to a food processor. Add the olive oil, Bone Broth, lemon juice, and sea salt.

4. Blend on high for about 30 seconds. Check the seasoning and adjust the salt to taste. Serve chilled.

## note

ROASTED FENNEL HUMMUS WILL KEEP FOR UP TO 5 DAYS, STORED IN AN AIRTIGHT CONTAINER IN THE REFRIGERATOR.

## ingredients

2 medium fennel bulbs (about 1 pound, or 450 g), diced into ½-inch (1 cm) pieces

1 medium white sweet potato (about 8 ounces, or 225 g), peeled and diced into ½-inch (1 cm) pieces

3 large cloves garlic, chopped

2 tablespoons (30 ml) extra virgin olive oil, plus extra for greasing the pan

3 tablespoons (45 ml) Bone Broth (page 34)

½ tablespoon (7 ml) lemon juice

½ teaspoon fine sea salt

## prep time
10 minutes

## cook time
40 minutes

## yield
2 cups (470 ml)

# RAINBOW VEGGIE WRAPS

HERE IS AN EASY, AIP-FRIENDLY LUNCH THAT DOESN'T REQUIRE A LOT OF PREPARATION—PERFECT FOR BUSY WORKDAYS, PICNICS, AND HIKES. USE THE RECIPE AS A TEMPLATE AND GET CREATIVE. MISSING CUCUMBERS IN THERE? ADD THEM. DON'T LIKE SCALLIONS? SKIP THEM. MAKE IT YOUR OWN BY SWAPPING OUT WHICHEVER INGREDIENTS YOU DON'T LIKE IN FAVOR OF THOSE YOU LIKE BEST. IT'S YOUR WRAP—ENJOY IT!

### ingredients

2 large collard green leaves

2 sheets nori

⅔ cup (150 g) Spicy Guacamole (page 39) or Strawberry-Beet Salsa (page 37)

⅔ cup (70 g) shredded carrots

6 slices cooked bacon

1 avocado, peeled, pitted, and sliced

2 scallions, chopped

Chopped fresh cilantro

Lime juice

Fine sea salt

### directions

1. To assemble the wraps: Lay the collard green leaves flat on 2 separate plates, followed by a sheet of nori on top.

2. Spread the Spicy Guacamole or Strawberry-Beet Salsa onto the wraps, then follow with the shredded carrots.

3. Add the bacon, avocado, and scallions. Sprinkle with cilantro, drizzle with lime juice, and season with a pinch of sea salt.

4. Roll the wraps as tightly as possible, cut in half, and serve.

### prep time
10 minutes

### yield
2 servings

### notes

NORI IS THE NAME FOR THE EDIBLE SEAWEED SHEETS OFTEN USED IN SUSHI.

IF YOU ARE MAKING THESE VEGGIE WRAPS TO GO, DON'T CUT THEM. LEAVE THEM WHOLE AND WRAP THEM TIGHTLY IN A PIECE OF ALUMINUM FOIL. KEEP REFRIGERATED UNTIL READY TO EAT.

*The Autoimmune Protocol Made Simple Cookbook*

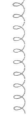

# COCKTAIL CHEESE BITES

ARE YOU NERVOUS ABOUT GIVING UP CHEESE IN ORDER TO COMPLY WITH AIP? I KNOW HOW THAT FEELS. THE GOOD NEWS IS, I HAVE DISCOVERED A LITTLE WORK-AROUND INVOLVING NUTRITIONAL YEAST, WHICH IMPARTS A CHEESY TASTE HERE. IT'S JUST THE THING TO SATISFY THAT CRAVING WE ALL KNOW SO WELL. SERVE THESE LITTLE BITES AT YOUR NEXT PARTY, AS A SNACK, OR EVEN IN A LUNCH BOX.

## directions

1. Place the oven rack in the middle position of the oven and preheat it to 350°F (175°C). Line a baking sheet with parchment paper and set aside.

2. Combine all the ingredients in a food processor. Process on high for about 30 seconds, until you obtain a smooth paste.

3. Scoop out 22 small portions with a spoon and form into 1-inch (2.5 cm) balls with your hands. Arrange the balls on the baking sheet so they don't touch.

4. Bake for about 18 minutes, until golden. Serve hot with Garlic-Lemon Mayonnaise or Ranch Dressing.

## notes

THESE COCKTAIL CHEESE BITES WILL KEEP FOR UP TO 5 DAYS IN THE REFRIGERATOR.

WARM UP SLOWLY ON A PARCHMENT-LINED BAKING SHEET IN THE OVEN AT 350°F (175°C) BEFORE SERVING.

### ingredients

1 cup (200 g) cooked spaghetti squash

½ cup (60 g) arrowroot flour

⅓ cup (40 g) coconut flour

1 teaspoon fine sea salt

1 teaspoon garlic powder

⅓ cup (40 g) nutritional yeast

3 tablespoons (45 ml) melted palm shortening

Garlic-Lemon Mayonnaise or Ranch Dressing (page 40 or 44)

### prep time
15 minutes

### cook time
18 minutes

### yield
22 bites

# DAIRY-FREE ZUCCHINI CHEESE

## ingredients

2 small zucchini
(about 12 ounces, or 340 g),
peeled and diced

½ cup (120 ml) water

2 tablespoons (30 ml)
melted coconut oil

2 teaspoons (10 ml)
lemon juice

¾ teaspoon fine sea salt,
or more to taste

4 tablespoons (36 g)
unflavored gelatin powder

1 tablespoon (8 g)
nutritional yeast (optional)

½ cup (30 g) minced
fresh parsley

## prep time
15 minutes

## cook time
5 minutes

## yield
2 cups (480 ml)

CHEESE IS ONE OF LIFE'S SMALL PLEASURES. WITH THIS ZUCCHINI-BASED TREAT, YOU DON'T HAVE TO FEEL DEPRIVED. PLUS, IT IS SO VERSATILE. YOU CAN SLICE IT, SHRED IT, AND MELT IT OVER ANY WARM PREPARATION, INCLUDING ROASTED VEGETABLES.

## directions

1. Steam the zucchini until tender (see Notes), about 5 minutes. Drain and allow the zucchini to cool a bit.

2. Add the zucchini, water, coconut oil, lemon juice, and sea salt to a blender and mix on high for 30 seconds, or until smooth.

3. Add the gelatin and nutritional yeast (if using). Blend for another 15 seconds. Pour the mixture into a bowl. Add the parsley and mix thoroughly.

4. Pour the preparation into a glass or ceramic container. Refrigerate for about 4 hours, until firm. Slice and serve with apple slices and Onion-Basil Crackers (page 29) or use as you would traditional cheese.

## notes

TO STEAM ZUCCHINI: PLACE A VEGETABLE STEAMER IN A POT, ADD 1 TO 2 INCHES (2.5 TO 5 CM) OF WATER, AND BRING TO A BOIL. ADD THE DICED ZUCCHINI, COVER, AND STEAM FOR ABOUT 5 MINUTES, UNTIL TENDER.

THE STEAMED ZUCCHINI WILL KEEP FOR UP TO 5 DAYS IN THE REFRIGERATOR AND THE ZUCCHINI CHEESE WILL KEEP FOR UP TO 7 DAYS IN THE REFRIGERATOR.

*The Autoimmune Protocol Made Simple Cookbook*

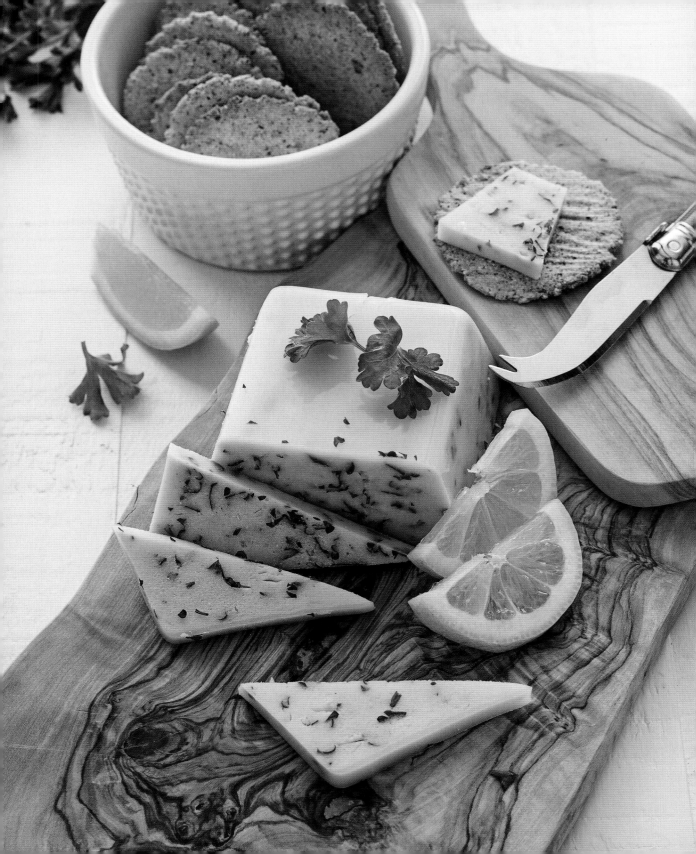

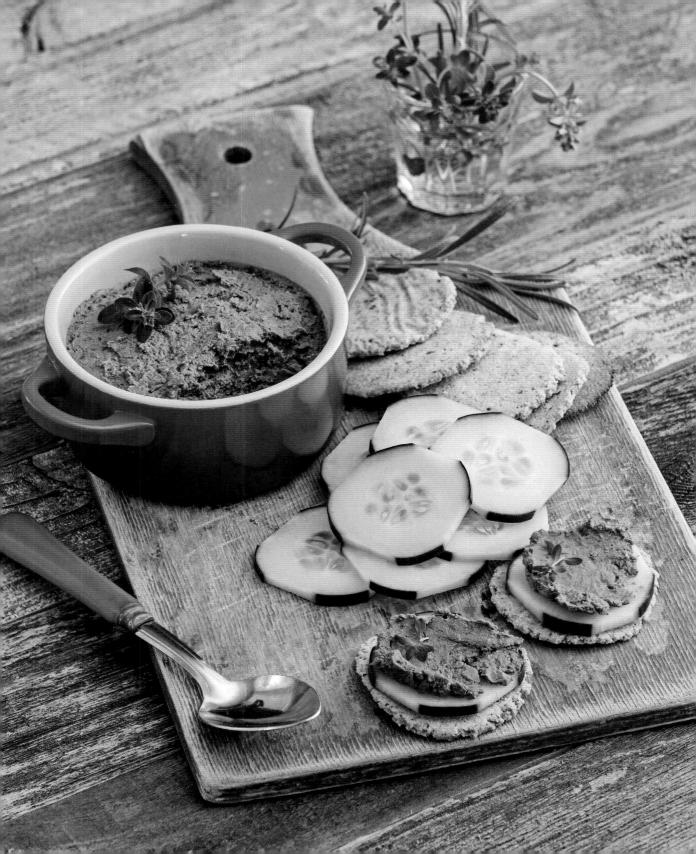

# BEGINNER'S LIVER PÂTÉ

LIVER IS AN ORGAN MEAT, OR OFFAL, AND IT'S A NUTRITIONAL POWERHOUSE THAT PLAYS AN IMPORTANT ROLE IN THE AUTOIMMUNE PROTOCOL. BEFORE YOU TURN THE PAGE THINKING YOU DON'T LIKE LIVER, KNOW THAT THIS VERSION IS BEGINNER-FRIENDLY. THERE ARE SO MANY COMPLEMENTARY FLAVORS AT PLAY HERE: THE SWEETNESS OF APPLES AND SWEET POTATOES, THE RICH AND EARTHY TANG OF LIVER, AND THE ENTICING AROMA OF ROSEMARY AND THYME. IT IS PERFECT FOR FIRST-TIME TESTERS.

## directions

1. Wash the liver and pat dry. Trim away the white sinew with a paring knife. Chop the liver into 1/2-inch (1 cm) pieces.

2. Heat the bacon fat in a large skillet over medium heat until thoroughly melted. Add the apple, sweet potato, shallot, and apple cider vinegar. Cover and cook, stirring occasionally, until the vegetables soften, about 10 to 12 minutes.

3. Add the liver, thyme, rosemary, and sea salt. Continue to cook uncovered, stirring frequently, for 6 to 8 minutes, until the liver is cooked through but still slightly pink inside. Remove from the heat and allow to cool.

4. Transfer the mixture to a blender or food processor, making sure to include all the cooking juices, and blend until smooth and creamy. You may have to do this in two batches. Check the seasoning and adjust the salt to taste.

5. Transfer the pâté to small lidded containers and refrigerate until needed.

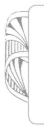

## notes

LARD MAY BE SUBSTITUTED FOR BACON FAT.

LIVER PÂTÉ WILL KEEP IN THE REFRIGERATOR FOR UP TO 5 DAYS. IT ALSO FREEZES WELL.

## ingredients

1 pound (450 g) chicken or beef liver

1/3 cup (80 ml) bacon fat

1 green apple, peeled, cored, and finely chopped

3/4 cup (100 g) peeled and finely chopped white sweet potato

1/2 cup (80 g) minced shallot

2 tablespoons (30 ml) apple cider vinegar

2 1/2 teaspoons (4 g) dried thyme

2 teaspoons (1 g) dried rosemary

1 teaspoon fine sea salt

## prep time
20 minutes

## cook time
20 minutes

## yield
2 1/3 cups (550 ml)

# CURRY CHICKEN SALAD

EVER WONDER WHAT TO DO WITH LEFTOVER CHICKEN BREASTS? CHICKEN SALAD IS ALWAYS A GOOD IDEA. THIS CURRIED VERSION IS RICH AND FULL OF WONDERFUL SPICES. EAT IT ON ITS OWN OR WRAP IT IN A COLLARD GREEN LEAF (OR AN AIP-APPROVED TORTILLA) AND CALL IT A CURRY BURRITO. THIS SALAD IS SO DELICIOUS, YOU COULD EVEN JUST SPREAD IT ON A SLICE OF ROSEMARY AND THYME FOCACCIA (PAGE 31). YOUR CALL.

## *ingredients*

2 cups (280 g) cooked and diced chicken

1 cup (120 g) finely sliced celery

1 red apple, diced

3 scallions, thinly sliced

2 tablespoons (21 g) golden raisins

¾ cup (175 ml) coconut yogurt

½ teaspoon turmeric powder

¼ teaspoon garlic powder

¼ teaspoon dried ground ginger

¼ teaspoon onion powder

¼ teaspoon fine sea salt, or more to taste

Pinch of ground cinnamon

Pinch of ground cloves

## *prep time*
15 minutes

## *yield*
5 servings

## *directions*

1. Mix the chicken, celery, apple, scallions, and raisins in a large bowl.

2. Mix the coconut yogurt, turmeric powder, garlic powder, ginger, onion powder, sea salt, cinnamon, and ground cloves in a small bowl until thoroughly combined.

3. Pour the sauce over the chicken mixture and mix well. Check the seasoning and adjust the salt to taste. Refrigerate until ready to serve.

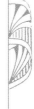

## *note*

SOME COCONUT YOGURTS ARE THICK AND DRY TASTING. ADD A LITTLE BIT OF COCONUT MILK OR WATER TO MAKE THE MIXTURE SMOOTHER AND CREAMIER IF YOU NEED TO.

*The Autoimmune Protocol Made Simple Cookbook*

# MEDITERRANEAN TUNA SALAD

OH, THE THINGS YOU CAN DO WITH A CAN OF TUNA! ADD SOME CUCUMBER FOR EXTRA CRUNCH, PLUMP AND SMOOTH KALAMATA OLIVES, TANGY CAPERS, AND RICH GARLIC FOR A FULL-BODIED AND SATISFYING MEDITERRANEAN TAKE ON A CLASSIC TUNA SALAD. SERVE THIS TUNA SALAD ON BUTTER LETTUCE CUPS AT YOUR NEXT LUNCHEON.

## directions

1. Place all the ingredients in a mixing bowl. Toss to combine, breaking up large chunks of tuna with a fork if necessary. Season with sea salt to taste.

2. Add more Mayonnaise to taste for a creamier consistency. Serve chilled.

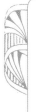

## notes

VARIATION: REPLACE THE MAYONNAISE WITH MASHED-UP AVOCADO AND A DASH OF LEMON JUICE OR USE EXTRA VIRGIN OLIVE OIL FOR A LIGHTER SALAD.

THIS SALAD WILL KEEP FOR UP TO 5 DAYS, STORED IN AN AIRTIGHT CONTAINER IN THE REFRIGERATOR.

### ingredients

2 (5-ounce, or 142 g) cans water-packed tuna, drained

½ English cucumber, peeled, seeded, and cut into ¼-inch (6 mm) pieces

⅓ cup (45 g) kalamata olives, finely sliced

3 tablespoons (45 ml) Mayonnaise (page 38), or more to taste

2 scallions, finely sliced

2 tablespoons (8 g) minced fresh parsley

1 tablespoon (9 g) capers

1 clove garlic, minced

Fine sea salt to taste

### prep time
10 minutes

### yield
3 cups (700 g)

# CHAPTER SEVEN

# SOUPS AND SALADS

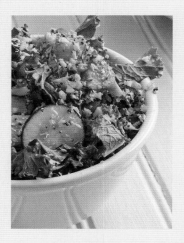

**ONE OF THE CORE PRINCIPLES** of the Autoimmune Protocol is nutrient density. Nutrients are essential for good health, and they can be found in spades in many vegetables. There isn't really an upper limit to the number of vegetables you can eat; just avoid all nightshade vegetables during the strict elimination phase of the Autoimmune Protocol (see page 19), though as you progress through the protocol, you may find that you can add some of them back in during the reintroduction phase.

Raw, steamed, cooked, or roasted, vegetables (and fruit) are excellent sources of vitamins, minerals, fibers, and antioxidants. They feed the beneficial bacteria in your gut, improving immune function, energy levels, and mental well-being. It might seem odd at first, but try to add vegetables to every meal, including breakfast, to maximize your intake.

It's important to remember that along with our mouths, we also eat with our eyes. You will be more apt to eat an attractive meal. The recipes in this chapter are designed to add maximum variety and color to your plate.

Each soup recipe will yield at least 4 or 5 servings, and many of them can be frozen. Each salad recipe can be served as a side dish to your main meal or eaten on its own. Add a source of protein, such as leftover cooked chicken or a few shrimp, to turn these salads into a complete meal. Or better yet, pair them with a bowl of vegetable-laden soup to double up on the veggies.

Welcome to AIP Soups and Salads.

# DANDELION-ZOODLE SALAD

HAVE YOU TASTED DANDELION LEAVES BEFORE AND FOUND THEM BITTER? I URGE YOU TO GIVE THEM ANOTHER TRY WITH THIS SEEMINGLY SIMPLE LITTLE SALAD. IT IS PACKED WITH NUTRIENTS AND NATURAL ANTIOXIDANTS FROM A POTENT MIX: AVOCADO + BLUEBERRIES + DANDELION GREENS = NUTRIENT PARTY! PLUS, THE RICH AND CREAMY SAUCE WILL KEEP YOU SATIATED FOR HOURS. SERVE WITH TEX-MEX MARINATED STEAK (PAGE 119) OR SEARED TUNA TATAKI (PAGE 142) FOR A NUTRIENT-DENSE MEAL.

## directions

1. Combine the zucchini noodles, dandelion leaves, blueberries, and red onion in a large bowl.

2. Place the avocados, olive oil, coconut milk, lemon juice, and sea salt in a blender or food processor. Blend until you obtain a smooth and creamy consistency.

3. Add the avocado sauce to the salad right before serving.

## note

TO MAKE ZUCCHINI NOODLES, OR ZOODLES: CUT OFF THE TOP AND BOTTOM OF THE ZUCCHINI AND CUT INTO NOODLES WITH A VEGETABLE SPIRALIZER. DON'T HAVE A SPIRALIZER? USE A VEGETABLE PEELER TO SLICE THE ZUCCHINI INTO THIN RIBBONS.

## ingredients

8 ounces (225 g) raw zucchini noodles (see Note)

3 ounces (85 g) chopped dandelion leaves

6 ounces (170 g) blueberries

2 ounces (55 g) sliced red onion

2 avocados, peeled and pitted

5 tablespoons (75 ml) extra virgin olive oil or avocado oil

2 tablespoons (30 ml) full-fat coconut milk

1 tablespoon (15 ml) lemon juice

¼ teaspoon fine sea salt

## prep time
10 minutes

## yield
4 servings

# JICAMA-MANGO SALAD

THIS SALAD IS WONDERFUL ON ITS OWN OR WITH GRILLED FISH OR MEAT. THE SWEETNESS OF THE MANGO, THE TARTNESS OF THE LIME JUICE, AND THE CRISPNESS OF THE JICAMA COME TOGETHER TO FORM A REFRESHING AND UPLIFTING COMBINATION. THIS SALAD DOESN'T KEEP WELL, SO IT IS BEST TO CONSUME IT SHORTLY AFTER YOU PREPARE IT.

## *ingredients*

1 small jicama
(about 1 pound, or 450 g)

1 small cucumber
(about 12 ounces, or 340 g)

1 large mango

½ packed cup (8 g) finely
chopped cilantro

2 scallions, finely chopped

Juice of 2 limes

Citrus Vinaigrette (page 45)

## *prep time*
20 minutes

## *yield*
4 to 6 servings

## *directions*

1. Peel and julienne the jicama. Cut off both ends of the cucumber and thinly slice. Peel, pit, and julienne the mango. You can speed up the process by using a mandoline slicer with a julienne blade.

2. Mix the jicama, cucumber, mango, cilantro, scallions, and lime juice in a large bowl. Refrigerate until needed. Add the dressing just before serving.

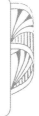

## *note*

JICAMA-MANGO SALAD
WILL KEEP FOR UP TO 2 DAYS
IN THE REFRIGERATOR.

*The Autoimmune Protocol Made Simple Cookbook*

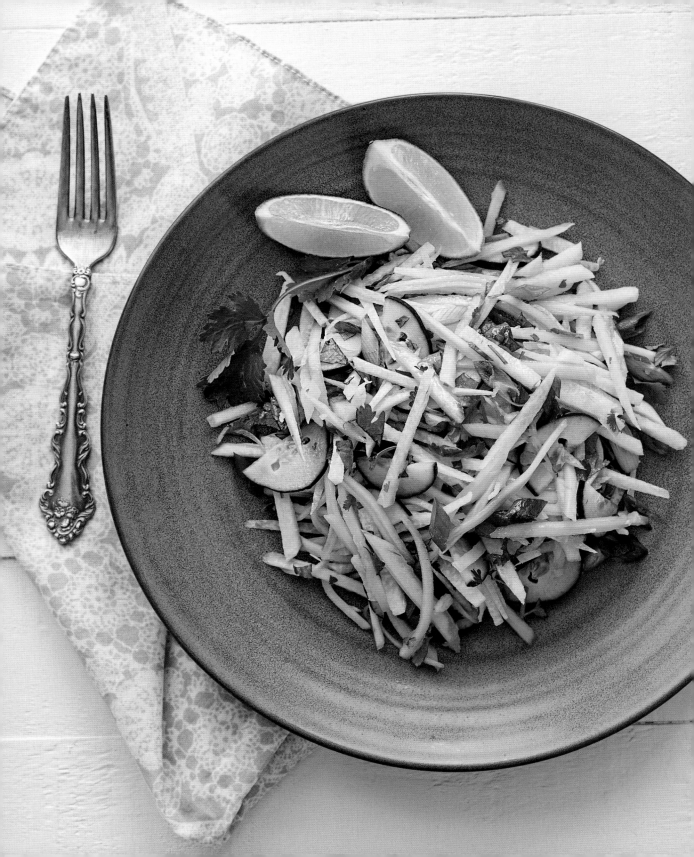

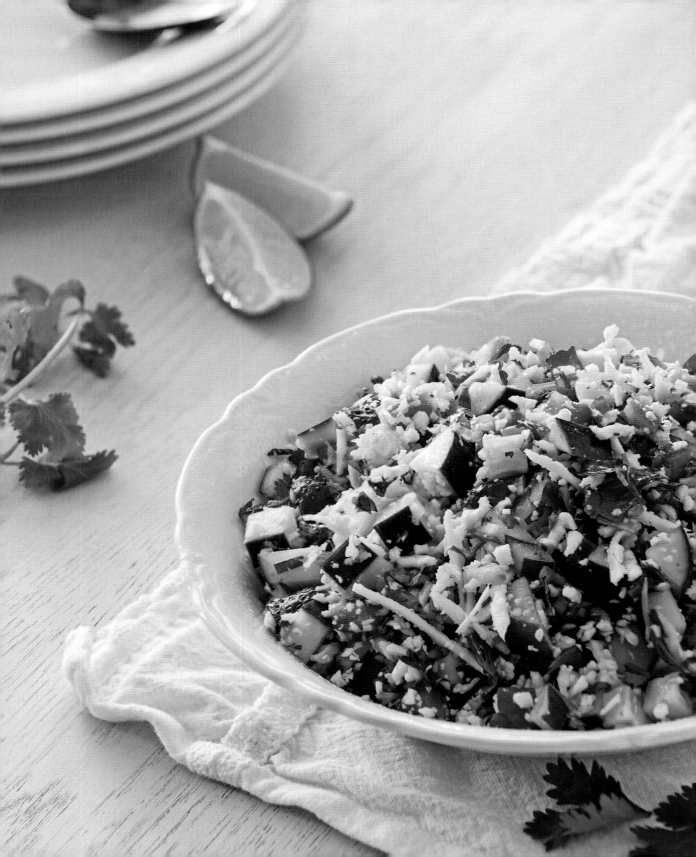

# REFRESHING CAULI-TABBOULEH

THIS WONDERFULLY INVIGORATING CAULIFLOWER TABBOULEH
HITS THAT COVETED SWEET SPOT BETWEEN DELICIOUS AND
HEALTHY. THE FRESH HERBS ADD A MAJOR BURST OF FLAVOR AND
ARE ALSO FULL OF VITAMINS AND ANTIOXIDANTS. DON'T HESITATE
TO EXPERIMENT WITH OTHER HERBS, SUCH AS MINT OR ITALIAN
PARSLEY. TRY YOUR FAVORITES!

## directions

1. Mix the cauliflower rice, strawberries, cucumber, red onion, scallions, parsley, cilantro, and sea salt in a large bowl.

2. Refrigerate until needed. Add the dressing right before serving.

## ingredients

2 cups (200 g)
raw Cauliflower Rice
(see page 106)

⅓ pound (150 g)
strawberries, hulled and cut
into ¼-inch (6 mm) pieces

1 small cucumber (about
8 ounces, or 225 g), cut into
¼-inch (6 mm) pieces

½ cup (60 g)
finely chopped red onion

2 scallions, finely chopped

½ cup (30 g)
minced fresh parsley

½ cup (8 g) minced
fresh cilantro

½ teaspoon fine sea salt

Citrus Vinaigrette (page 45)

## prep time
15 minutes

## yield
4 servings

## note

UNDRESSED, TABBOULEH WILL KEEP
FOR UP TO 5 DAYS IN AN AIRTIGHT
CONTAINER IN THE REFRIGERATOR.

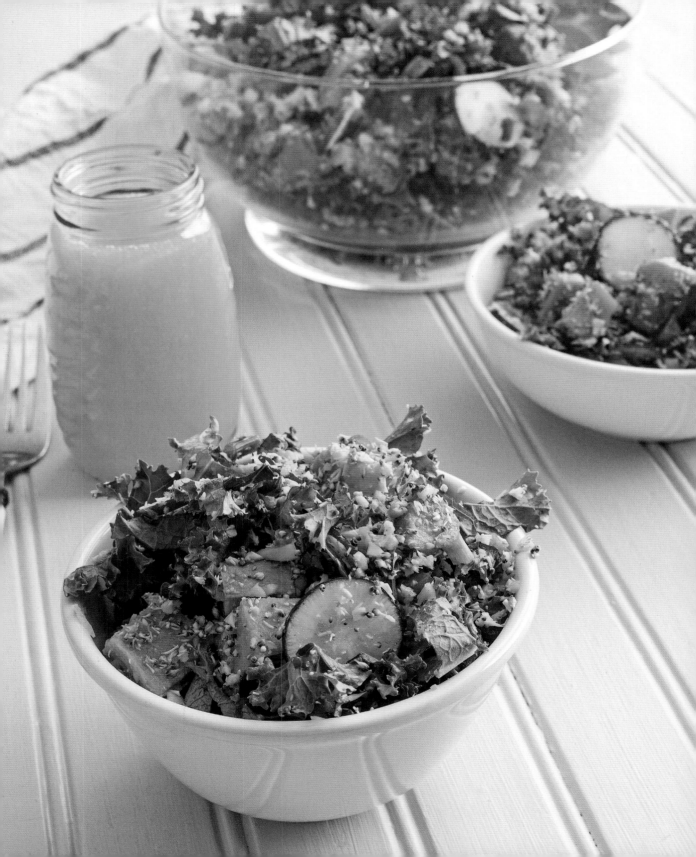

# ANTIOXIDANT KALE SALAD

YOU MAY BE A LITTLE OVER KALE, BUT I ASSURE YOU, THIS ANTIOXIDANT-RICH, NUTRIENT-PACKED SALAD WILL BRING YOU RIGHT BACK INTO KALE'S CORNER. FEEL FREE TO ADD SOME PROTEIN FOR A FULL MEAL. IF RAW VEGGIES AREN'T YOUR THING, YOU MAY WANT TO BLANCH THE KALE FOR A FEW MINUTES (SEE NOTES). IT WILL TENDERIZE THE LEAVES JUST ENOUGH.

## *directions*

1. Mix the kale, sweet potatoes, broccoli rice, scallions, and radishes in a large bowl.

2. Add the dressing right before serving.

## *notes*

TO MAKE BROCCOLI RICE: CUT UP BROCCOLI INTO PIECES, TRANSFER TO A FOOD PROCESSOR, AND, USING A STANDARD S-SHAPED BLADE, CHOP/PULSE UNTIL YOU OBTAIN SMALL GRAINS. I PREFER TO PROCESS FLORETS AND STALKS IN TWO SEPARATE BATCHES.

IF YOU CHOOSE TO BLANCH THE GREEN VEGGIES FOR THIS SALAD, BRING A LARGE POT OF WATER TO A RAPID BOIL. SALT THE WATER IF DESIRED. ADD THE VEGGIES TO THE BOILING WATER AND COOK FOR 30 TO 60 SECONDS. AFTER COOKING, IMMEDIATELY PLUNGE THE VEGGIES INTO A BOWL OF ICE WATER. WHEN COOL, DRAIN THE VEGGIES AND PREPARE THE SALAD AS ABOVE.

## *ingredients*

⅓ pound (225 g) kale, stemmed and thinly sliced

1 pound (450 g) cooked sweet potatoes, peeled and diced

2 cups (200 g) raw broccoli rice (see Notes)

5 scallions, finely chopped

10 radishes, thinly sliced

Citrus Vinaigrette (page 45), Creamy Cilantro Dressing (page 44), or Chimichurri Verde (page 43)

## *prep time*
20 minutes

## *yield*
4 servings

# MIXED VEGGIE BOWL

WHEN YOU HAVE ALL THE INGREDIENTS READY, THIS VEGGIE BOWL TAKES ONLY A FEW MINUTES TO PUT TOGETHER. WITH THAT IN MIND, COOK THE CAULIFLOWER RICE AND BEETS IN ADVANCE (EVEN THE DAY BEFORE). BOTH WILL KEEP WELL IN THE FRIDGE. THIS DISH WORKS PERFECTLY FOR A WARM-WEATHER LUNCH OR LIGHT EVENING MEAL. AN ADDITION OF CHILLED, COOKED SHRIMP WOULDN'T GO AMISS, EITHER.

### ingredients

2 cups (250 g) cooked
Speedy Cauliflower Rice
(page 106)

2 cups (220 g)
shredded carrots

2 cups (270 g)
diced cucumber

2 cups (340 g)
diced cooked beets

2 avocados, peeled,
pitted, and sliced

1 cup (30 g) broccoli sprouts

Fine sea salt, to taste

Citrus Vinaigrette (page 45),
Creamy Cilantro Dressing
(page 44), or Mayonnaise
(page 38)

### directions

1. Divide the ingredients evenly among 4 bowls in the following order: cauliflower rice at the bottom, carrots, cucumber, beets, and avocados. Garnish with the broccoli sprouts on top.

2. Season with sea salt to taste and drizzle with your favorite dressing.

### prep time
15 minutes

### cook time
20 minutes

### yield
4 servings

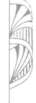

### note
TRY REPLACING THE DICED COOKED BEETS WITH STRAWBERRY-BEET SALSA (PAGE 37).

*The Autoimmune Protocol Made Simple Cookbook*

# BABY ARUGULA AND ROOT VEGETABLE SALAD

THERE IS SOMETHING SO HOMEY ABOUT A ROASTING PAN FILLED WITH SWEET, TENDER ROASTED VEGGIES. I ALWAYS PICTURE THEM IN AUTUMN BECAUSE THEY ARE WARM AND FILLING, BUT HONESTLY, I LOVE AND CRAVE THEM IN EVERY SEASON. THIS RECIPE IS SO SIMPLE, YOU CAN THROW IT TOGETHER AFTER A LONG DAY WHEN YOU'RE TOO TIRED TO COOK, BUT STILL WANT SOMETHING HEALTHY AND DELICIOUS.

## *directions*

1. Place the oven rack in the middle position of the oven and preheat it to 350°F (175°C).

2. Mix the butternut squash, red onion, olive oil, oregano, and sea salt in a large, rimmed roasting pan. Spread in a single layer.

3. Roast, stirring a few times while cooking, for about 40 minutes, until the vegetables are tender. Let the vegetables cool and then mix in the arugula.

4. Add the dressing right before serving.

## *ingredients*

1 pound (450 g) butternut squash, cut into ½-inch (1 cm) pieces

1 small red onion (about 8 ounces, or 225 g), cut fajita style (see Note)

2 tablespoons (30 ml) extra virgin olive oil

½ tablespoon (3 g) dried oregano

½ teaspoon fine sea salt

4 ounces (115 g) baby arugula

Citrus Vinaigrette (page 45) or Creamy Cilantro Dressing (page 44)

## *prep time*
15 minutes

## *cook time*
40 minutes

## *yield*
4 servings

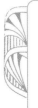

## *note*

TO SLICE A RED ONION "FAJITA STYLE," CUT IT IN HALF LENGTHWISE (FROM STEM TO STEM). PLACE THE HALVED ONION CUT-SIDE DOWN ON A CUTTING BOARD. RUN A SHARP KNIFE FROM STEM TO STEM, MAKING ¼-INCH (6 MM) SLICES FROM ONE SIDE OF THE ONION TO THE OTHER.

# TURMERIC-GINGER SOUP

THIS SOUP SCREAMS AUTOIMMUNE PROTOCOL. IT CONTAINS BOTH TURMERIC AND GINGER—A DOUBLE WHAMMY OF HEALING BENEFITS. BOTH ARE POWERFUL ANTIOXIDANTS, BOTH CONTAIN POWERFUL ANTI-INFLAMMATORY PROPERTIES, AND BOTH ADD A DELICIOUS BURST OF FLAVOR TO THIS WARMING SOUP. IT'S QUITE LITERALLY THE PERFECT SOUP FOR WHEN YOU ARE FEELING A BIT UNDER THE WEATHER.

*ingredients*

1½ pounds (680 g) carrots, peeled and chopped

1 pound (450 g) sweet potatoes, peeled and chopped

1 yellow onion (about 8 ounces, or 225 g), chopped

1 (1-inch, or 2.5 cm) knob fresh ginger, peeled and sliced

1 (1-inch, or 2.5 cm) knob fresh turmeric, peeled and sliced

1½ quarts (1.5 L) Bone Broth (page 34)

1 cup (240 ml) full-fat coconut milk

Fine sea salt, to taste

## *directions*

1. Place the carrots, sweet potatoes, onion, ginger, turmeric, and Bone Broth in a large stockpot.

2. Bring to a boil over high heat. Reduce the heat to medium and cook, covered, for about 20 minutes, until the vegetables are tender.

3. Remove from the heat and blend with an immersion blender until smooth.

4. Stir in the coconut milk and season to taste with sea salt.

*prep time*
15 minutes

*cook time*
20 minutes

*yield*
5 (2-cup, or 480 ml) servings

*notes*

THIS SOUP WILL KEEP FOR UP TO 5 DAYS, STORED IN AN AIRTIGHT CONTAINER IN THE REFRIGERATOR.

FREEZES WELL.

# JULIENNE VEGETABLE SOUP

THIS GORGEOUS SOUP IS AN EXCELLENT WAY TO ADD MORE VEGETABLES TO YOUR DIET. A DELICIOUS BLEND OF GARDEN-FRESH VEGETABLES, IT IS VERY SIMPLE TO PREPARE AND FULL OF VITAMINS AND FIBER. ADD COOKED CHICKEN OR SHRIMP FOR AN EXTRA SOURCE OF PROTEIN. BESIDE THE FACT THAT THE JULIENNE CUT IS VERY STYLISH, IT ALSO ENSURES THAT VEGETABLES COOK RAPIDLY AND EVENLY ALL THE WAY THROUGH—A WIN-WIN!

## directions

1. Cut the carrots, celery, and turnips into 2- to 3-inch (5 to 7.5 cm) pieces with a sharp knife, then thinly slice lengthwise. Flip the pieces on their sides and slice again to obtain even matchsticks. You can speed this process by using a mandoline slicer with a julienne blade.

2. Thinly slice the leeks, rinse in cold water, and drain.

3. Place the vegetables and Bone Broth in a large stockpot and bring to a boil over high heat. Reduce the heat to medium and cook, covered, for 12 to 15 minutes, until the vegetables are tender, but not mushy.

4. Add the cilantro and season to taste with sea salt.

### ingredients

8 ounces (225 g) carrots, peeled

8 ounces (225 g) celery

8 ounces (225 g) turnips, peeled

8 ounces (225 g) leeks

2 quarts (2 L) Bone Broth (page 34)

½ cup (8 g) finely chopped fresh cilantro

Fine sea salt, to taste

### prep time
20 minutes

### cook time
15 minutes

### yield
6 (2-cup, or 480 ml) servings

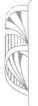

## notes

A SQUEEZE OF LEMON ADDS A HIT OF BRIGHTNESS.

THIS SOUP WILL KEEP FOR UP TO 5 DAYS, STORED IN AN AIRTIGHT CONTAINER IN THE REFRIGERATOR.

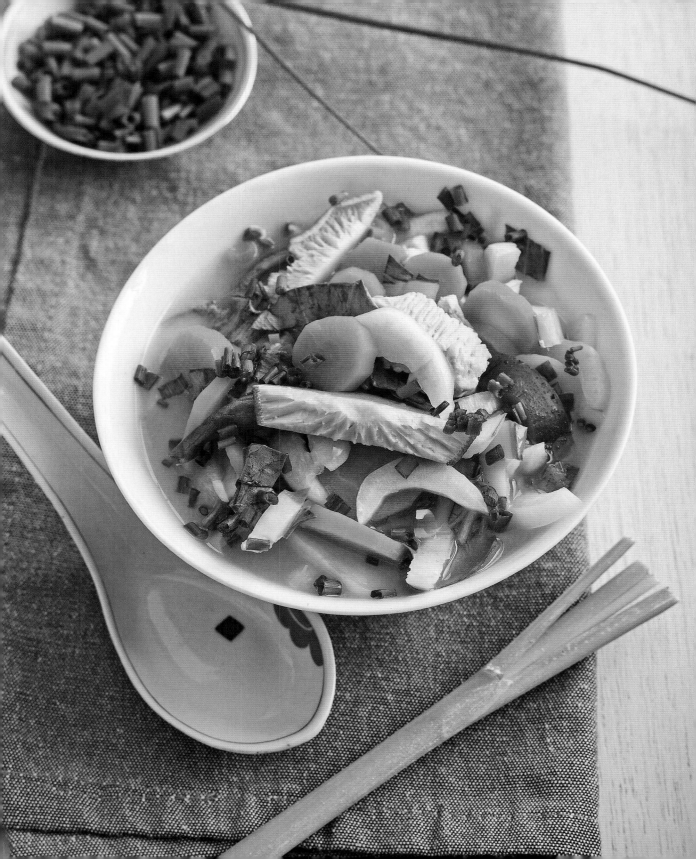

# LEMONGRASS CHICKEN SOUP

LEMONGRASS'S FRESH SCENT HAS MADE IT POPULAR AS AN ESSENTIAL OIL. IN THAT FORM, IT IS RUMORED TO BE BENEFICIAL IN AIDING UPSET STOMACHS AND HEADACHES AS WELL AS BOOSTING ENERGY. HERE, IT IS A WONDERFULLY FRAGRANT ADDITION TO CHICKEN SOUP THAT TAKES IT FROM COMFORTABLE TO EXCEPTIONAL.

## directions

1. Place the shiitake mushrooms in a large bowl and cover with warm water. Soak for 20 minutes. Drain and slice into ¼-inch (6 mm) strips.

2. Bring the Bone Broth to a boil in a covered stockpot over high heat. Add the chicken, carrots, mushrooms, lemongrass, and sea salt. Reduce the heat to medium and cook for 25 minutes.

3. Add the bok choy and continue to cook, covered, for 5 minutes.

4. Remove from the heat and stir in the coconut milk and coconut aminos. Check the seasoning and adjust the salt to taste.

5. Serve hot with a garnish of minced chives.

## note

THIS SOUP WILL KEEP FOR UP TO 5 DAYS, STORED IN AN AIRTIGHT CONTAINER IN THE REFRIGERATOR.

## ingredients

1 ounce (30 g) dehydrated shiitake mushrooms (about 15 pieces)

2 quarts (2 L) Bone Broth (page 34)

1 pound (450 g) skinless chicken breasts, cut into bite-size pieces

12 ounces (340 g) thinly sliced carrots

2 small stalks lemongrass, thinly sliced

1½ teaspoons (9 g) fine sea salt

12 ounces (340 g) chopped baby bok choy

½ cup (120 ml) full-fat coconut milk

1 tablespoon (15 ml) coconut aminos

Minced fresh chives, for garnish

### prep time
20 minutes

### cook time
25 minutes

### yield
6 (2-cup, or 480 ml) servings

# WHITE MINESTRONE

MINESTRONE SOUP, WITH ITS RICH, TOMATOEY BROTH, STARCHY POTATOES, AND TINY DITALINI IS THE STUFF OF DREAMS, BUT TOMATOES, POTATOES, AND PASTA (NO MATTER HOW TINY) ARE NOT ALLOWED WITH AIP. NEVER FEAR! YOU DON'T HAVE TO GIVE UP THE WARMTH AND DELICIOUSNESS OF THIS CLASSIC SOUP. THIS AIP MINESTRONE IS HEARTY, RICH, FULL OF SATISFYING ROOT VEGGIES, AND SURE TO WARM YOUR BELLY. SERVE WITH A PIECE OF ROSEMARY AND THYME FOCACCIA (PAGE 31).

## ingredients

6 ounces (170 g) bacon, sliced

12 ounces (340 g) carrots, peeled and diced

8 ounces (225 g) yellow onion, finely chopped

8 ounces (225 g) parsnips, peeled and diced

8 ounces (225 g) sweet potatoes, peeled and diced

2 tablespoons (5 g) minced fresh thyme

1½ quarts (1.5 L) Bone Broth (page 34)

Fine sea salt, to taste

## prep time
15 minutes

## cook time
26 minutes

## yield
5 (2-cup, or 480 ml) servings

## directions

1. Cook the bacon, stirring frequently, in a stockpot over medium-high heat, for about 6 minutes, until golden but not crispy.

2. Transfer the bacon with a slotted spoon to a paper towel–lined plate. Reserve the bacon fat in the pot.

3. Add the carrots, onion, parsnips, sweet potatoes, and thyme to the pot. Mix well and sauté, stirring frequently, for 5 minutes over medium-high heat.

4. Add the Bone Broth. Bring to a boil over high heat. Reduce the heat to medium and cook, covered, for about 15 minutes, until the vegetables are tender.

5. Add the bacon back to the pot and season to taste with sea salt.

## notes

MAKE THIS MINESTRONE EXTRA NUTRITIOUS BY ADDING FRESH AVOCADO TO YOUR BOWL.

IT'S A GREAT RECIPE FOR BATCH COOKING, AS IT FREEZES WELL.

THIS SOUP WILL KEEP FOR UP TO 5 DAYS, STORED IN AN AIRTIGHT CONTAINER IN THE REFRIGERATOR.

*The Autoimmune Protocol Made Simple Cookbook*

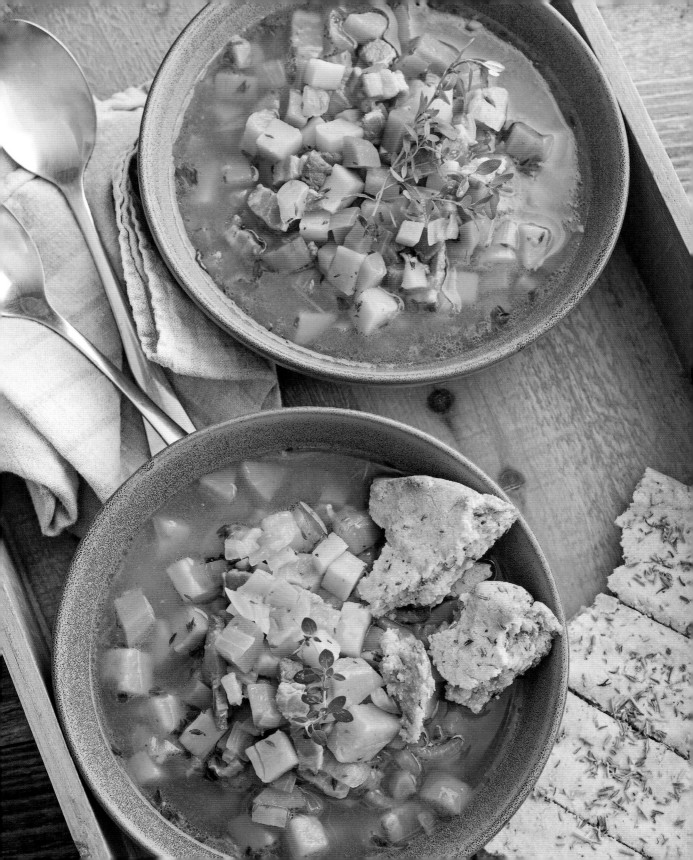

# CREAM OF PARSNIP SOUP

I BELIEVE THAT PARSNIPS ARE CRIMINALLY UNDERUSED. LIKE THEIR CLOSE COUSIN THE CARROT, PARSNIPS ARE SWEET AND VERSATILE. ROASTED, STEAMED, MASHED, OR SAUTÉED, PARSNIPS BLOOM WITH JUST A LITTLE ATTENTION. HERE, I'VE CREATED A COMFORTING AND EASY-TO-PREPARE SOUP THAT WILL KEEP YOU WARM ON A COOL EVENING. FOR AN EVEN MORE SATISFYING MEAL, ADD A LITTLE PROTEIN, SUCH AS SHREDDED BEEF OR CHICKEN.

### ingredients

2 pounds (900 g) parsnips, peeled and chopped

12 ounces (340 g) cauliflower florets, chopped

2 slices uncured bacon (about 3 ounces, or 85 g), sliced

2 quarts (2 L) Bone Broth (page 34)

½ cup (120 ml) full-fat coconut milk

Fine sea salt to taste

### prep time
10 minutes

### cook time
20 minutes

### yield
6 (2-cup, or 480 ml) servings

### directions

1. Place the parsnips, cauliflower, bacon, and Bone Broth in a large stockpot. Bring to a boil over high heat. Reduce the heat to medium and cook, covered, for about 20 minutes, until the vegetables are tender.

2. Remove from the heat and blend with an immersion blender until smooth.

3. Stir in the coconut milk and season to taste with sea salt.

### notes

CREAM OF PARSNIP SOUP WILL KEEP IN THE REFRIGERATOR FOR UP TO 5 DAYS IN AN AIRTIGHT CONTAINER.

FREEZES WELL.

*The Autoimmune Protocol Made Simple Cookbook*

# RUSTIC CHARD AND BACON SOUP

SOME THINGS ARE HARD TO GET OVER. FIRST LOVES COME TO MIND. ADD THIS RUSTIC, COMFORTING SOUP TO YOUR LIST OF UNFORGETTABLE EVENTS. THE EARTHY CHARD AND THE RICH BACON DON'T HAVE TO WORK TOO HARD TO IMPRINT THEMSELVES ON YOUR PALATE. YOU CAN TRY, BUT I'M BETTING YOU WON'T FORGET THIS SOUP ANYTIME SOON.

## directions

1. Heat the olive oil in a stockpot over medium-high heat. Add the bacon, onion, and garlic. Sauté, stirring constantly, for about 5 minutes, until slightly golden.

2. Add the turnips and Bone Broth. Bring to a boil, then reduce the heat to medium and cook, covered, for about 25 minutes, until the vegetables are tender.

3. Add the chard and continue to cook for 5 minutes.

4. Serve hot with thick pieces of Rosemary and Thyme Focaccia (page 31).

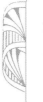

## note

THIS SOUP WILL KEEP FOR UP TO 5 DAYS, STORED IN AN AIRTIGHT CONTAINER IN THE REFRIGERATOR.

## ingredients

3 tablespoons (45 ml) extra virgin olive oil

3 slices bacon (4½ ounces, or 135 g), thinly sliced

1 yellow onion (about 8 ounces, or 225 g), thinly chopped

4 cloves garlic, minced

2 turnips (about 1½ pounds, or 675 g), diced

1½ quarts (1.5 L) Bone Broth (page 34)

1 bunch chard (about 1 pound, or 450 g), stemmed and thinly sliced

## prep time
20 minutes

## cook time
35 minutes

## yield
5 (2-cup, or 480 ml) servings

# CHAPTER EIGHT

# VEGETABLES

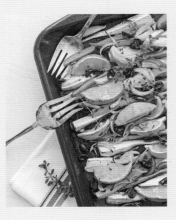

**HAVE YOU EVER STOPPED** to consider the true wealth of vegetables available to us? Grocery stores, health food stores, and farmers' markets all over the country overflow with an incredible selection of vegetables (and fruits) all year long. This chapter will help you take full advantage of this bounty.

Aside from the nightshade vegetables (see page 19) that we avoid on AIP, all vegetables are allowed. Aim for three-fourths of your plate to be filled with a colorful and varied assortment of high- and low-starch vegetables. Take advantage of the changing seasons to vary your vegetable intake and maybe try something new.

Food quality is also important. Go for organic, locally grown produce when you can. If this isn't possible, don't let it deter you from continuing your AIP journey! You have much to gain from adding fresh produce to your diet, even if it is not organic.

Note that many recipes in this chapter are meant to help you swap your old favorites for healthier, AIP-approved versions. Here are a few examples:

* Swap French fries for yuca fries.
* Swap pasta for baked spaghetti squash or vegetable noodles.
* Swap rice for cauliflower rice.
* Swap mashed potatoes for mashed broccoli.

A bonus is that all these recipes are also great for batch cooking and freezing. You can make a large batch on the weekend when you have more time, then freeze them for later in the week when you're tired and in need of a fast addition to dinner.

Welcome to AIP Vegetables.

# BAKED SPAGHETTI SQUASH

THE FIRST TIME I TASTED SPAGHETTI SQUASH, I WAS SHOCKED AT
HOW SWEET IT WAS. MANY SQUASH VARIETIES HAVE A NATURAL
SWEETNESS, BUT THIS WAS SOMETHING ELSE. SOMETHING
DELICIOUS! I LOVE TO MATCH THAT SWEETNESS WITH THE BITE
OF GARLIC AND THE TANG OF FRESH PARSLEY. SERVE THIS BAKED
SQUASH HOT WITH ROASTED MEAT OR EXPERIMENT WITH USING IT
IN "PASTA" SALAD.

## directions

1. Place the oven rack in the middle position of the oven and preheat to 400°F (200°C).

2. Cut off the top and bottom of the spaghetti squash with a serrated knife. Slice it in half lengthwise. Scoop out the seeds and discard. Place both halves, cut-side down, in a baking dish and add 1 inch (2.5 cm) water.

3. Bake for about 30 minutes, until the skin softens and gives a little when you push it with your finger. Do not overcook or the flesh will be too mushy.

4. Transfer the spaghetti squash to a plate, cut-side up, with a large slotted spatula. Let the squash cool a little bit before scraping out the flesh with a fork, making spaghetti noodles.

5. Heat the coconut oil in a large skillet over medium heat. Add the onion and garlic and sauté, stirring frequently, for about 10 minutes, until tender. Add the spaghetti squash noodles and parsley, and mix thoroughly.

6. Season with sea salt to taste. Serve hot.

## note

SERVE WITH MEATBALLS (PAGE 123), VERSATILE
PULLED PORK CARNITAS (PAGE 126), BEEF-BISON
BURGERS (PAGE 127), OR RUSTIC MEATLOAF
(PAGE 130).

## ingredients

1 spaghetti squash
(2½ to 3 pounds,
or 1.1 to 1.4 kg)

2 tablespoons (30 ml)
coconut oil

1 yellow onion
(about 8 ounces, or 225 g),
finely chopped

4 cloves garlic, minced

¾ cup (45 g) minced
fresh parsley

Fine sea salt to taste

### prep time
15 minutes

### cook time
40 minutes

### yield
4 to 5 servings

# CRISPY YUCA FRIES

YUCA FRIES, ALSO KNOWN AS CASSAVA FRIES, ARE VERY POPULAR IN LATIN AMERICA AND ARE A GREAT ALTERNATIVE TO TRADITIONAL FRENCH FRIES. USE EITHER FRESH OR FROZEN YUCA ROOTS. DON'T SKIP THE PARBOILING, AS IT WASHES OFF THE EXCESS STARCH AND BREAKS DOWN THE TOUGH FLESH OF THIS ROOT. FIND YUCA ROOT AT YOUR LOCAL HEALTH FOOD OR ETHNIC FOOD STORE.

*ingredients*

2 pounds (900 g) yuca roots (if frozen, let thaw completely)

¼ cup (60 ml) melted coconut oil

Fine sea salt, to taste

Garlic-Lemon Mayonnaise (page 40) or Chimichurri Verde (page 43)

*prep time*
10 minutes

*cook time*
30 minutes

*yield*
5 to 6 servings

## directions

1. Cut off the ends of the yuca roots and peel with a knife or a vegetable peeler. Cut the roots into ¼- to ½-inch (6 mm to 1 cm)-thick fries, leaving out the tough fibrous core. (If using previously frozen yuca, the core has already been removed.) Rinse.

2. Place the yuca fries in a large pot and fill with water until 1 inch (2.5 cm) above fries. Bring to a boil over high heat. Reduce the heat to medium and cook, covered, for about 10 minutes, until fork tender.

3. Meanwhile, place the oven rack in the top third of the oven and preheat it to 400°F (200°C).

4. Drain the fries and pat dry with paper towels. Toss with the coconut oil and sea salt. Arrange the fries on 1 or 2 rimmed baking sheets, ensuring they don't touch.

5. Bake, turning the fries over halfway through, for about 30 minutes, until golden. Serve hot with Garlic-Lemon Mayonnaise or Chimichurri Verde.

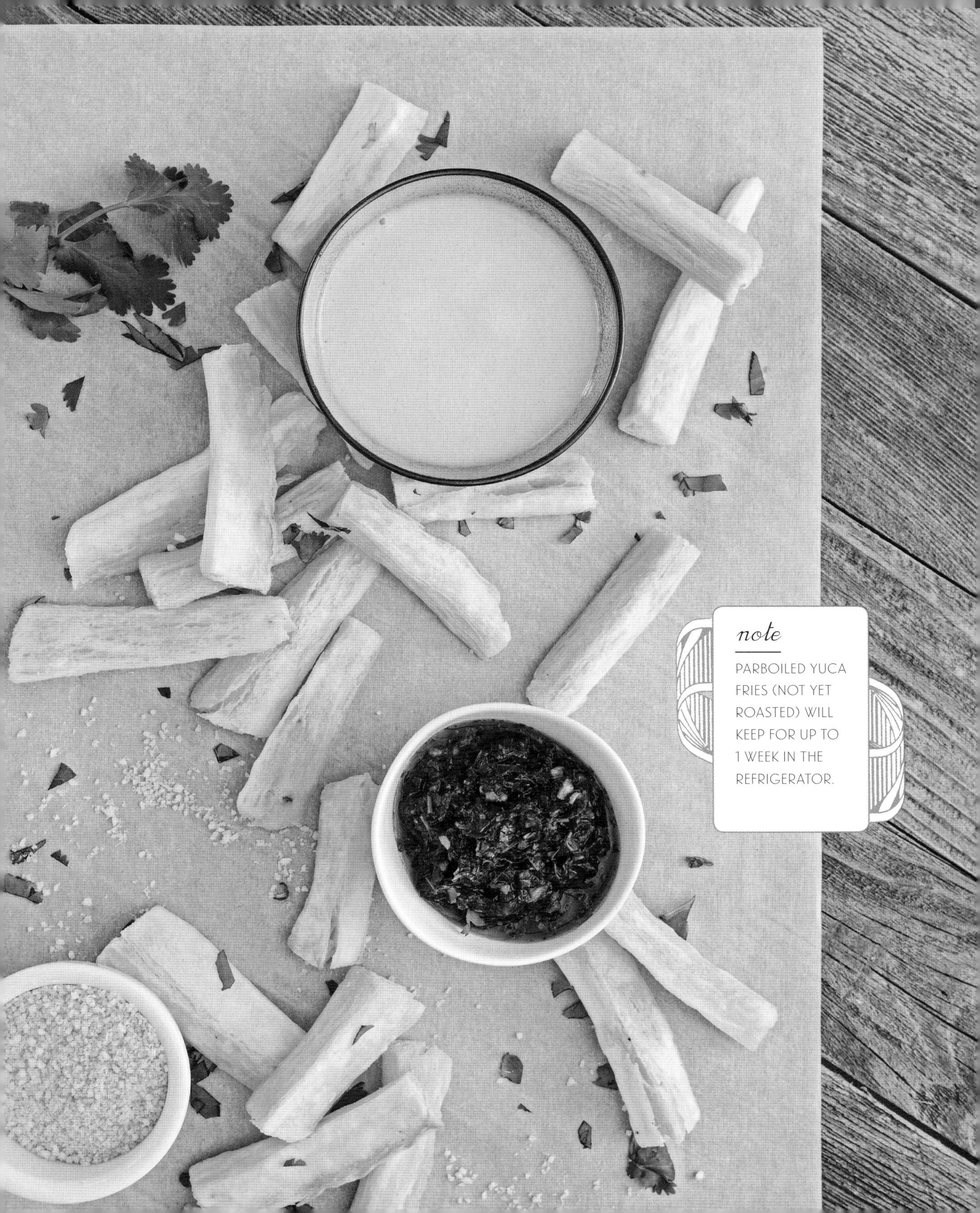

*note*

PARBOILED YUCA FRIES (NOT YET ROASTED) WILL KEEP FOR UP TO 1 WEEK IN THE REFRIGERATOR.

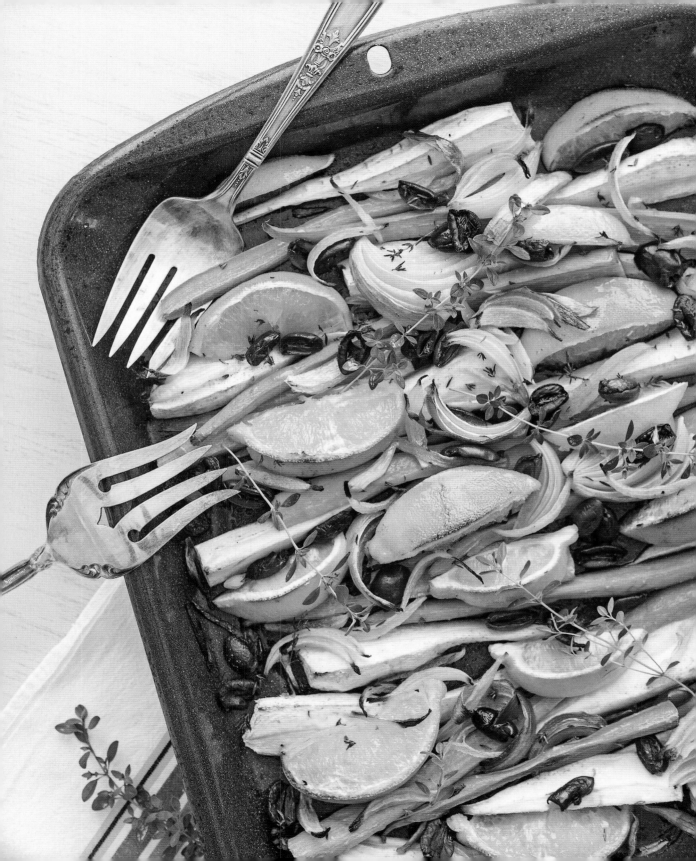

# ROASTED ROOT VEGETABLES AND CITRUS

ROASTING BRINGS OUT THE NATURAL SWEETNESS OF MOST VEGETABLES AND ENHANCES THE DEPTH OF FLAVOR TO A DEGREE OTHERWISE UNNOTICED. HERE, I ROAST MY VEGGIES WITH CHUNKS OF CITRUS FOR A NICE HIT OF ACID TO BRIGHTEN THE RICHNESS OF THE CARROTS AND PARSNIPS. SERVE WITH ROASTED CHICKEN OR PORK AND A SALAD FOR A COLORFUL AND NUTRIENT-DENSE MEAL.

## directions

1. Place the oven rack in the middle position and preheat it to 400°F (200°C).

2. Combine the carrots, parsnips, lemon wedges, orange wedges, and red onion on a shallow rimmed roasting pan.

3. Scatter the olives and thyme on top. Drizzle with the coconut oil and season with the sea salt.

4. Roast until the vegetables are tender, about 45 minutes, stirring halfway through.

5. When the vegetables are done, squeeze the cooked citrus pieces over the vegetables (carefully, as they will be hot), then discard. Toss to evenly distribute the juice. Serve hot with your favorite roasted or grilled meat.

## ingredients

12 ounces (340 g) carrots, peeled and cut lengthwise

12 ounces (340 g) parsnips, peeled and cut lengthwise

1 lemon, unpeeled, cut into 8 pieces

1 orange, unpeeled, cut into 8 pieces

1 small red onion (about 5 ounces, or 140 g), cut fajita style (see Note on page 91)

½ cup (65 g) chopped kalamata olives

Handful fresh thyme, roughly chopped

2 tablespoons (30 ml) melted coconut oil

1 teaspoon fine sea salt

## prep time
15 minutes

## cook time
45 minutes

## yield
4 to 5 servings

# SPEEDY CAULIFLOWER RICE

YOU CAN SERVE CAULIFLOWER WITH PRETTY MUCH ANYTHING, WHICH MAKES CAULIFLOWER RICE THE PERFECT ALTERNATIVE TO REGULAR RICE AND OTHER GRAINS, SUCH AS MILLET AND QUINOA. EAT IT RAW IN A DELICIOUS AND REFRESHING CAULI-TABBOULEH (PAGE 87), OR LIGHTLY COOKED AND SEASONED TO YOUR LIKING. AS AN ADDED BONUS, IT REHEATS EXCEPTIONALLY WELL.

## *ingredients*

1 head cauliflower
(about 2 pounds, or 1.1 kg)

2 tablespoons (30 ml) extra
virgin olive oil or coconut oil

4 large chard leaves,
stemmed and thinly sliced

⅓ cup (6 g)
chopped fresh cilantro

Fine sea salt to taste

## *prep time*
10 minutes

## *cook time*
10 minutes

## *yield*
5 to 6 servings

## *directions*

1. Discard all the green leaves, then core and cut up the cauliflower into small florets.

2. Transfer the florets to a food processor equipped with an S-shaped blade and chop/pulse until the florets turn into small grains. You may have to do this in several batches.

3. Heat the olive oil in a large skillet over medium heat. Add the cauliflower rice and cook, uncovered and stirring frequently, for 8 to 10 minutes, until tender. Don't let it get mushy!

4. Remove from the heat, add the chard and cilantro, and mix well. Season with sea salt to taste.

## *notes*

GIVE SOME FLAVOR TO YOUR CAULIFLOWER RICE BY ADDING FRESH GINGER, TURMERIC POWDER, OR SAFFRON.

STORE RAW OR COOKED CAULIFLOWER IN AN AIRTIGHT CONTAINER IN THE REFRIGERATOR FOR UP TO 5 DAYS.

# CREAMY MASHED BROCCOLI

DON'T BE FOOLED BY THE APPARENT SIMPLICITY OF THIS DISH.
RICH, CREAMY, AND REMINISCENT OF THE COMFORT FOOD OF
OUR YOUTH, THIS MASHED BROCCOLI IS A MASTERPIECE IN
DISGUISE. IT'S A MUST TO BRIGHTEN UP A GRAY DAY THIS WINTER.
OF COURSE, THERE'S NO RULE THAT SAYS YOU CAN'T EAT IT IN
SUMMER AND SPRING, TOO. IF IT WERE UP TO ME, BROCCOLI
WOULD BE ON THE MENU EVERY DAY OF THE YEAR.

## directions

1. Trim the broccoli, remove the tough outer skin from the stalks, and chop.
   Peel the sweet potato, remove any eyes or brown spots, and chop.

2. Place a vegetable steamer in a pot, add 1 to 2 inches (2.5 to 5 cm) water, and
   bring to a boil over medium-high heat. Add the broccoli and sweet potato,
   cover, and steam for 10 to 15 minutes, until tender. Let cool for a few minutes.

3. Combine the broccoli, sweet potato, and coconut milk in a blender or food
   processor and blend on low speed for about 30 seconds, until creamy. You
   may have to do this in several batches.

4. Season to taste with sea salt and garnish with fresh parsley before serving.

### ingredients
1 pound (450 g) broccoli

1 white sweet potato
(about 8 ounces, or 225 g)

½ cup (120 ml) full-fat
coconut milk

Fine sea salt, to taste

Minced fresh parsley,
for garnish

### prep time
15 minutes

### cook time
15 minutes

### yield
3 cups (700 g)

## note

I RECOMMEND THIS RECIPE FOR BATCH
COOKING, AS IT ALSO FREEZES WELL.
THAW AND REHEAT SLOWLY OVER
MEDIUM-LOW HEAT ON THE STOVETOP.

# COLESLAW

THIS COLORFUL AND REFRESHING COLESLAW PACKS A PUNCH.
IT'S THE PERFECT NUTRITIOUS SIDE DISH FOR YOUR NEXT PICNIC
OR POTLUCK. THE APPLE AND FRESH LIME JUICE REALLY BRIGHTEN
UP THE FLAVOR PROFILE OF THIS DECEPTIVELY TAME DISH. IF YOU
ARE PREPARING IT IN ADVANCE, ADD THE DRESSING JUST BEFORE
SERVING TO PRESERVE FRESHNESS.

## *ingredients*

1 green apple, julienned

Juice of 1 lime

12 ounces (340 g) red
cabbage, thinly sliced

12 ounces (340 g) carrots,
peeled and shredded

4 scallions, thinly sliced

½ cup (8 g) minced fresh
cilantro or (30 g) parsley

1 (1-inch, or 2.5 cm)
knob fresh ginger,
peeled and grated

¼ cup (60 g) Mayonnaise
(page 38) or Garlic-Lemon
Mayonnaise (page 40),
or to taste

## *prep time*
15 minutes

## *yield*
5 to 6 servings

## *directions*

1. Toss the julienned apples with the lime juice in a small bowl, ensuring the apples are well coated. This will prevent oxidation.

2. Combine all the ingredients except the mayonnaise in a large bowl and mix well.

3. Add the mayonnaise right before serving. If you prefer moister coleslaw, add extra mayonnaise 1 tablespoon (12 g) at a time.

## *note*

SERVE WITH TEX-MEX MARINATED STEAK
(PAGE 119), BEEF-BISON BURGERS (PAGE 127),
PAN-FRIED FISH STICKS (PAGE 139), OR
GARLIC-SEAWEED SHRIMP (PAGE 147).

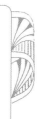

*The Autoimmune Protocol Made Simple Cookbook*

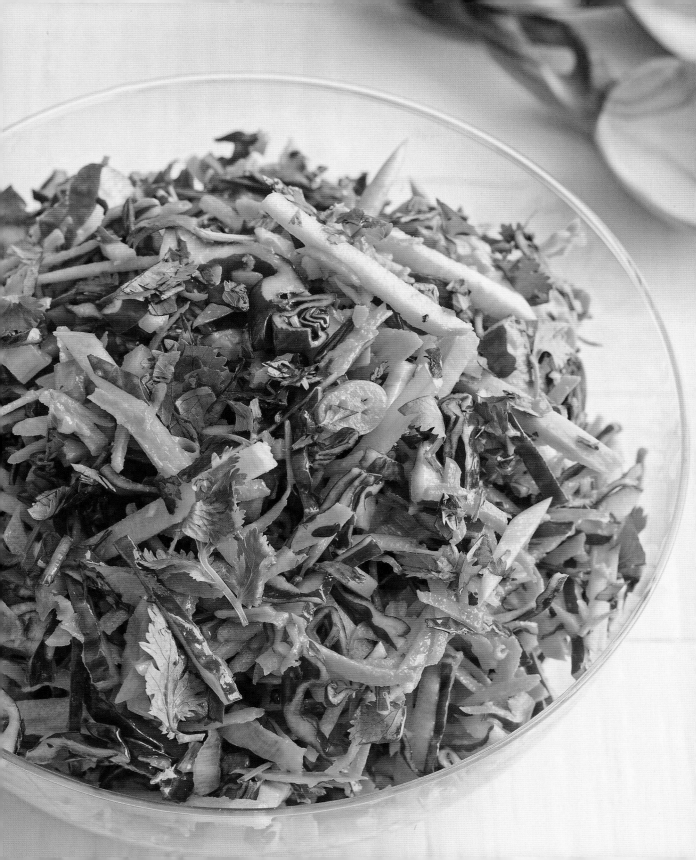

# VEGGIE TACOS

ONE OF THE BEST THINGS ABOUT TACOS IS HOW VERSATILE THEY ARE. YOU CAN FILL THEM WITH ANYTHING, REALLY. HERE, I'VE GATHERED UP SOME OF MY FAVORITE VEGETABLES TO CREATE A COLORFUL ARRAY OF TACOS THAT WILL CERTAINLY BOOST YOUR VEGGIE INTAKE FOR THE WEEK. I LOVE THE WAY THE TEXTURES OF THE COOKED AND RAW VEGGIES WORK TOGETHER. I KNOW YOU WILL PUT THESE TACOS ON REGULAR ROTATION AT YOUR HOUSE.

## *ingredients*

1¼ pounds (560 g) peeled and diced butternut squash

2 tablespoons (30 ml) extra virgin olive oil

½ teaspoon fine sea salt

½ teaspoon turmeric powder

8 No-Fail Turmeric Tortillas (page 32)

**SUGGESTED TACO TOPPINGS:**

4 cups (80 g) baby arugula

2½ cups (220 g) chopped red cabbage

1 recipe Strawberry-Beet Salsa (page 37)

½ cup (50 g) chopped scallion

½ cup (8 g) chopped fresh cilantro

Creamy Cilantro Dressing (page 44)

## *directions*

1. Place the oven rack in the middle position and preheat the oven to 400°F (200°C).

2. Combine the butternut squash, olive oil, sea salt, and turmeric powder in a large bowl. Stir well and spread in a single layer on a rimmed baking sheet.

3. Bake for 20 to 25 minutes, until the vegetables are tender and golden.

4. If the No-Fail Turmeric Tortillas are cool, reheat before serving. Arrange the other toppings in small dishes on the table.

5. Serve the roasted butternut squash in warm No-Fail Turmeric Tortillas with the toppings.

## *prep time*
20 minutes

## *cook time*
25 minutes

## *yield*
4 servings
(2 tortillas per person)

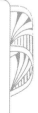

## *note*
TO MIX THINGS UP, SWAP THE BUTTERNUT SQUASH FOR SWEET POTATOES, ACORN SQUASH, OR PUMPKIN.

*The Autoimmune Protocol Made Simple Cookbook*

# CREAMED KALE

NUTRIENT DENSITY IS VERY IMPORTANT IF WE WANT TO PROVIDE OUR BODIES WITH ALL THE TOOLS NEEDED TO REPAIR AND HEAL. AND DARK LEAFY GREENS, RICH IN ANTIOXIDANTS AND POWERFUL ANTI-INFLAMMATORY PROPERTIES, ARE HIGH ON THE LIST OF NUTRIENT-DENSE FOODS. I LIKE TO COOK MINE LIGHTLY IN A LITTLE BIT OF COCONUT MILK TO SOFTEN THE STRONG, EARTHY TASTE.

## directions

1. Remove and discard the hard stem from the kale leaves. Chop the leaves.

2. Heat the olive oil in a large skillet over medium heat. Add the onion and sauté for 5 minutes. Add the kale and coconut milk and continue to cook, covered, stirring a few times, for another 5 minutes.

3. Season with sea salt to taste right before serving.

### ingredients

8 ounces (225 g) kale

3 tablespoons (45 ml) extra virgin olive oil

½ cup (60 g) finely chopped onion

½ cup (120 ml) full-fat coconut milk

Fine sea salt to taste

### prep time
10 minutes

### cook time
10 minutes

### yield
4 servings

## note

THIS RICH DISH MAKES AN EXCELLENT ACCOMPANIMENT TO FISH AND LIGHTER MEATS.

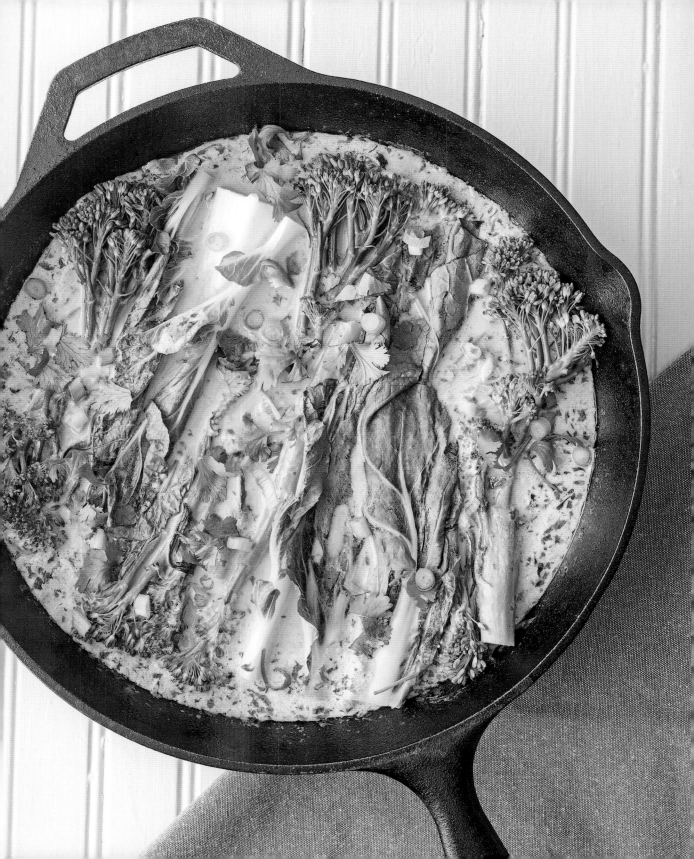

# VEGETABLE CURRY

IF YOU THOUGHT YOU COULDN'T HAVE A SATISFYING CURRY ON AIP, THINK AGAIN. THIS MOUTHWATERING CURRY IS ALL IN THE DETAILS. LEMONGRASS, GINGER, GARLIC, AND TURMERIC COME TOGETHER IN A BURST OF FLAVOR. DID YOU KNOW THAT COOKING TURMERIC WITH HEALTHY FATS UNLEASHES ITS FULL ANTI-INFLAMMATORY POTENCY? AS AN ADDED BONUS, THIS FABULOUS CURRY GOES BEAUTIFULLY WITH THAI BEEF (PAGE 129).

## directions

1. Place the lemongrass, ginger, garlic, cilantro, and lime juice in a food processor. Process until you obtain a crumbly and fragrant base. Set aside.

2. Melt the coconut oil in a large skillet over medium heat. Add the red onion and sauté for 5 minutes. Add the lemongrass mixture and cook, stirring continually, for another minute.

3. Whisk in the coconut milk, Bone Broth, turmeric powder, cinnamon, and sea salt.

4. Add the broccolini and cook, covered, for 10 minutes. Add the bok choy and cook, covered, for an additional 5 minutes, or until the vegetables are tender.

5. Check the seasoning and adjust the salt to taste. Serve with a garnish of cilantro and scallions.

## note

TRY REPLACING THE VEGETABLES WITH BROCCOLI, CAULIFLOWER, OR SWISS CHARD TO CHANGE THINGS UP.

## ingredients

1 stalk lemongrass, thinly sliced

1 (1-inch, or 2.5 cm) knob fresh ginger, peeled and sliced

2 large cloves garlic, sliced

1 packed cup (16 g) chopped fresh cilantro, plus extra for garnish

2 tablespoons (30 ml) lime juice

2 tablespoons (30 ml) coconut oil

½ cup (60 g) finely chopped red onion

1 (14-ounce, or 400 ml) can full-fat coconut milk

½ cup (120 ml) Bone Broth (page 34)

1 tablespoon (9 g) turmeric powder

½ teaspoon ground cinnamon

½ teaspoon fine sea salt

12 ounces (340 g) broccolini

12 ounces (340 g) bok choy, cut in half lengthwise

Chopped scallion, for garnish

### prep time
10 minutes

### cook time
25 minutes

### yield
4 servings

# SWEET POTATO GRATIN

BEFORE STARTING THE AIP, I WAS VERY FOND OF GRATINS. LOVELY, WARM, COMFORTING CASSEROLES THICK WITH CREAM AND CHEESE WERE MY FAVORITES—THINK POTATO GRATIN, BROCCOLI GRATIN, AND SEAFOOD GRATIN. THERE IS JUST NOTHING QUITE LIKE THEM—UNTIL NOW! WITH ITS LUSH POTATO FLAVOR AND RICH, CREAMY SAUCE, THIS SWEET POTATO GRATIN FILLS THAT "COMFORT FOOD" SPACE IN MY SOUL.

## *ingredients*

2 large sweet potatoes (about 1¾ pounds, or 800 g), peeled and thinly sliced

1 yellow onion (about 8 ounces, or 225 g), thinly sliced

1 teaspoon garlic powder

1 (14-ounce, or 400 ml) can full-fat coconut milk

3 tablespoons (24 g) nutritional yeast

1 tablespoon (15 ml) coconut aminos

1 teaspoon fine sea salt

Minced fresh thyme, for garnish

*prep time*
15 minutes

*cook time*
50 minutes

*yield*
4 to 6 servings

## *directions*

1. Place the oven rack in the middle position and preheat the oven to 400°F (200°C).

2. Arrange a layer of sweet potatoes on the bottom of a 6½ x 9-inch (16 x 23 cm) glass dish, followed by a layer of onions. Sprinkle with the garlic powder. Continue layering until you have used all the vegetables.

3. Stir the coconut milk, nutritional yeast, coconut aminos, and sea salt in a small bowl and pour evenly over the vegetables.

4. Bake for about 50 minutes, until the vegetables are tender.

5. Serve hot with a garnish of fresh thyme.

*note*

I RECOMMEND THIS RECIPE FOR BATCH COOKING. IT ALSO FREEZES WELL. THAW BEFORE REHEATING SLOWLY OVER MEDIUM-LOW HEAT ON THE STOVETOP.

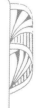

*The Autoimmune Protocol Made Simple Cookbook*

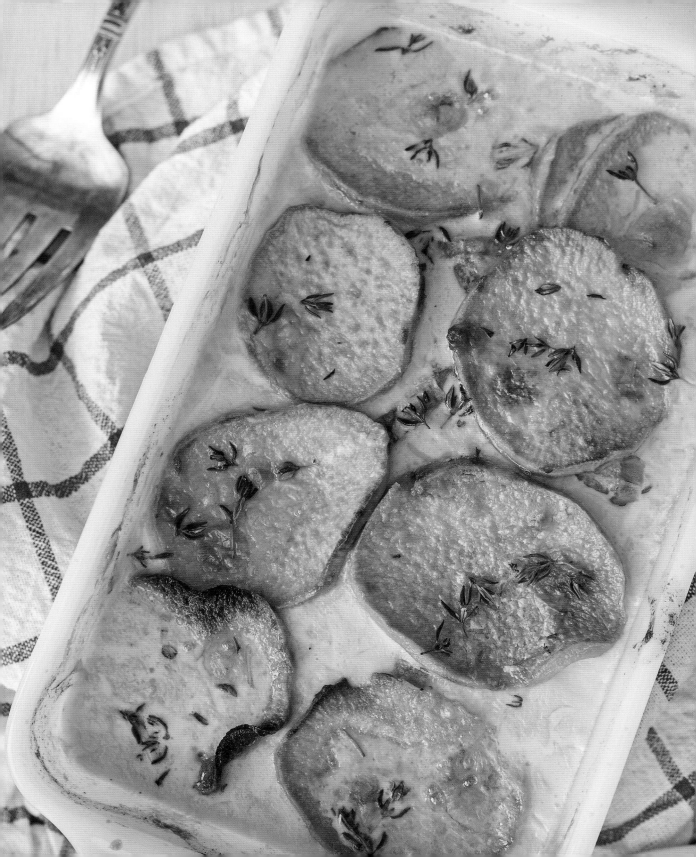

# BASIL ZUCCHINI NOODLES

DID YOU KNOW THAT YOU CAN TURN VEGETABLES INTO NOODLES WITH THE HELP OF A SPIRALIZER? IT'S TRUE! MY FAVORITE VEGETABLE TO USE IS ZUCCHINI. ZUCCHINI NOODLES HAVE A WONDERFULLY UNIQUE CREAMY/CRUNCHY TEXTURE THAT IS SO DELICIOUS AND JUST PERFECT FOR SAUCES. MAKE SURE YOU USE A LARGE SKILLET FOR THIS RECIPE, AS IT REQUIRES A LOT OF VEGGIES.

## ingredients

2 large zucchini
(about 1½ pounds, or 680 g)

3 tablespoons (45 ml)
extra virgin olive oil

8 ounces (225 g)
spinach leaves, chopped

Fine sea salt to taste

8 basil leaves, thinly sliced

Chimichurri Verde
(page 43) to taste

### prep time
10 minutes

### cook time
10 minutes

### yield
4 servings

## directions

1. Cut off the top and bottom of the zucchini and spiralize with a vegetable spiralizer or peeler (see Notes).

2. Heat the olive oil in a large skillet over medium heat. Add the zucchini noodles and spinach. Mix well. Cover and cook, stirring occasionally, for 8 to 10 minutes, until al dente. Add sea salt to taste.

3. Garnish with fresh basil and Chimichurri Verde right before serving.

## notes

IF YOU DON'T HAVE A VEGETABLE SPIRALIZER, YOU CAN USE A VEGETABLE PEELER TO PEEL THE ZUCCHINI INTO FLAT NOODLES, REMINISCENT OF TAGLIATELLE.

STORE RAW ZUCCHINI NOODLES IN THE REFRIGERATOR FOR UP TO 5 DAYS IN A RESEALABLE PLASTIC BAG LINED WITH A PAPER TOWEL.

*The Autoimmune Protocol Made Simple Cookbook*

# SIMPLE ROASTED TURNIPS

ROASTING IS A TECHNIQUE THAT CAN TAKE A HUMBLE INGREDIENT—A TURNIP, FOR INSTANCE—AND TURN IT INTO SOMETHING YOU CRAVE. THAT'S IMPORTANT WITH AIP, GIVEN THAT SO MUCH OF OUR DIET CONSISTS OF VEGETABLES. IT CAN GET BORING AFTER A WHILE. IT'S IMPORTANT TO TRY TO MIX IT UP A BIT. TRY THIS INCREDIBLY SIMPLE DISH WITH YOUR FAVORITE MEAT AND A FRESH SALAD FOR A WONDERFUL FAMILY MEAL.

## directions

1. Place the oven rack in the middle position and preheat the oven to 350°F (175°C).

2. Mix all the ingredients in a shallow rimmed roasting pan.

3. Roast, stirring a few times during cooking, for 40 to 50 minutes, until the turnips are tender and golden.

4. Serve hot with a drizzle of olive oil or refrigerate for later.

### ingredients

1¾ pounds (800 g) turnips, cut into ½-inch (1 cm) pieces

3 tablespoons (45 ml) extra virgin olive oil

1 tablespoon (1.5 g) minced fresh rosemary

¼ teaspoon fine sea salt, or more to taste

### prep time
10 minutes

### cook time
50 minutes

### yield
4 servings

## note

TRY SWAPPING TURNIPS FOR ANY OTHER ROOT VEGETABLE, SUCH AS CARROTS, BEETS, OR SWEET POTATOES. IF YOU DON'T HAVE FRESH ROSEMARY ON HAND, REPLACE WITH THYME OR TARRAGON.

# CHAPTER NINE

# MEAT-BASED MAIN DISHES

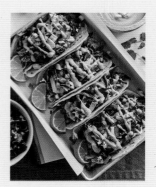

**HERE WE ARE AT THE HEART** of the matter: protein. Everyone talks about how much meat you will need to eat when adopting this lifestyle. The truth (as with so many things) lies somewhere in the middle. Yes, you will be consuming a healthy amount of meat, poultry, and seafood, but given the impressive versatility of protein, you will hardly feel as though you are overdoing it.

Just like vegetables (and fruit), meat is an important source of nutrients that you don't want to neglect as you focus on restoring your health. Quality is important. Budget permitting, try to consume organic, grass-fed, and pasture-raised meat and poultry. If this isn't an option for you right now, don't be concerned. Don't think for a second that you won't be able to achieve positive results with regular, nonorganic meat and poultry.

A good way to source healthy meat and poultry is to work with a local farmer in your area. Farmers are always happy to connect with appreciative customers, and many of them will sell directly to you via local farmers' markets. Your local farmers are also a fantastic source of bones for homemade bone broth and that other nutritional powerhouse, organ meat.

Pair any of the recipes in this chapter with a big salad or cooked vegetables (or both!) for a nutrient-filled meal. Many of these recipes are also great for batch cooking and suitable for freezing, which makes them great timesavers.

Welcome to AIP Meat-Based Main Dishes.

# TEX-MEX MARINATED STEAK

THIS MARINADE BRINGS A SATISFYING HIT OF FLAVOR TO ALMOST ANY MEAT WITHOUT BEING OVERPOWERING. THE TARTNESS OF LIME JUICE PAIRED WITH AN AROMATIC BOUQUET OF HERBS AND SPICES WILL WRING THE MOST FLAVOR OUT OF YOUR FOOD. IF YOU ARE FEELING ADVENTUROUS, WHY NOT CREATE YOUR OWN MARINADE? THERE ARE MANY INGREDIENTS TO CHOOSE FROM, EVEN ON AIP. (SEE PAGE 19.)

## directions

1. Place the meat in a resealable plastic bag.

2. To make the marinade: Mix the olive oil, lime juice, cilantro, oregano, cinnamon, garlic powder, and onion flakes in a bowl and pour over the meat.

3. Close the bag and massage the meat, making sure it is well coated with the marinade. Refrigerate for 2 hours, massaging now and again. Remove the steak from the refrigerator and bring to room temperature.

4. Heat a nonstick frying pan over medium-high heat until hot. Take the meat out of the bag and shake off the excess marinade. Place in the pan and cook for 3 to 4 minutes (depending on the thickness of the steak) on each side, until a brown crust has formed. You want the inside to remain pink. If using a stainless steel pan, you may have to add some oil to the pan before searing the meat so it doesn't stick to the pan too much.

5. Transfer the meat to a wooden cutting board, cover with aluminum foil, and let rest for 10 minutes.

6. Slice the steak across the grain and at an angle with a sharp chef's knife. Season with sea salt to taste and garnish with minced cilantro.

## note

OTHER POSSIBLE INGREDIENTS FOR MAKING YOUR OWN AIP MARINADE INCLUDE COCONUT AMINOS, MINCED ONION, SCALLION, MINCED GINGER, MINCED GARLIC, LEMONGRASS, AND TURMERIC.

### ingredients

1¼ pounds (565 g) beef flank steak

**FOR THE MARINADE:**

⅓ cup (80 ml) extra virgin olive oil or avocado oil

Juice of 1 lime

1 teaspoon dried cilantro

1 teaspoon dried oregano

½ teaspoon ground cinnamon

½ teaspoon garlic powder

½ teaspoon dried onion flakes

Fine sea salt, to taste

Minced fresh cilantro, for garnish

### prep time
5 minutes + 2 hours marinating

### cook time
8 minutes

### yield
4 servings

# HONEY-LIME CHICKEN WITH PEACH SALSA

8 large chicken drumsticks
(about 2 pounds, or 900 g)

**FOR THE MARINADE:**

½ cup (120 ml)
extra virgin olive oil

¼ cup (60 ml) honey

¼ cup (60 ml) lime juice

3 tablespoons (45 ml)
coconut aminos

¾ teaspoon fine sea salt

**FOR THE PEACH SALSA**
**(MAKES 3 CUPS, OR 700 G):**

4 peaches, peeled and finely
diced

1 large avocado, peeled,
pitted, and finely diced

4 scallions, finely chopped

⅓ cup (6 g) finely chopped
fresh cilantro

3 tablespoons (45 ml) lime
juice, plus more for serving

¼ teaspoon fine sea salt

*prep time*
20 minutes + 2 hours
marinating

*cook time*
40 minutes

*yield*
4 servings

FINGER-LICKING DELICIOUSNESS! THIS CHICKEN DELIVERS A BIG BURST OF FLAVOR THAT YOU WILL START DREAMING OF. AND THE SALSA! YOU WILL WANT TO SERVE THIS SALSA WITH JUST ABOUT EVERYTHING, AND THE GOOD NEWS IS, YOU CAN. TRY IT ON COCONUT YOGURT FOR A SWEET-SAVORY BREAKFAST TREAT OR OVER FISH FOR A SUMMERY DINNER OUT ON THE PATIO. DON'T EAT THE SPOON!

## directions

1. Place the chicken in a resealable plastic bag.

2. To make the marinade: Mix the olive oil, honey, lime juice, coconut aminos, and sea salt in a bowl. Pour over the chicken and seal the bag, turning it over a few times to coat the chicken completely.

3. Marinate in the refrigerator, turning the bag over a few more times during the process, for at least 2 hours, ideally overnight.

4. To make the Peach Salsa: Combine the peaches, avocado, scallions, cilantro, lime juice, and sea salt in a bowl. Mix well and refrigerate until needed.

5. Place the oven rack in the middle position and preheat the oven to 400°F (200°C).

6. Transfer the chicken to a shallow, rimmed roasting pan. Cover with leftover marinade. Roast, basting a few times, for 35 to 40 minutes, until the chicken is golden brown and cooked through to 165°F (74°C).

7. Serve immediately with a drizzle of lime juice and a side of Peach Salsa.

*note*

TO MAKE PREPARING
THE SALSA EASIER,
CHOOSE AVOCADOS
AND PEACHES THAT ARE
RIPE, BUT STILL FIRM.

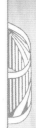

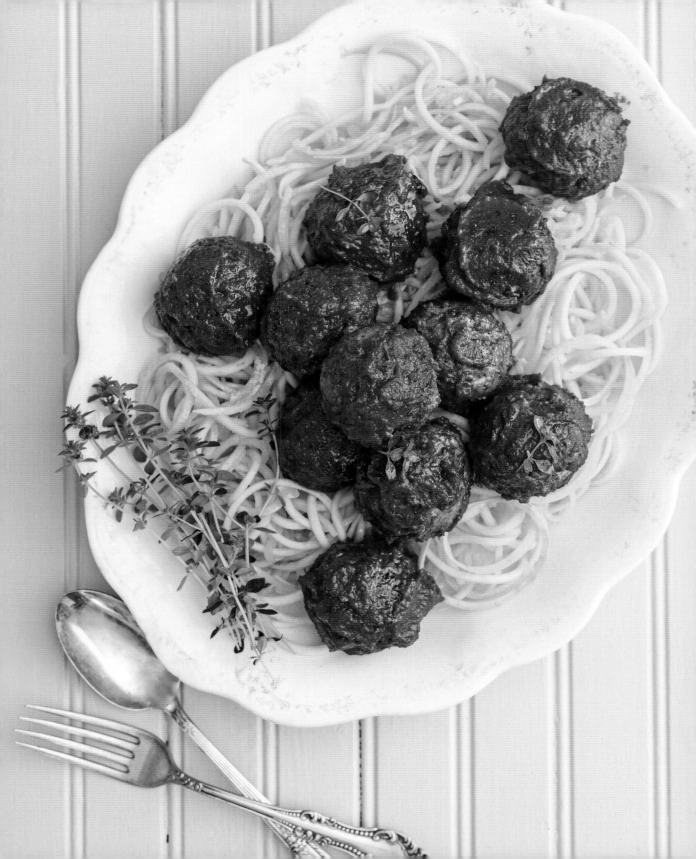

# MEATBALLS

PERFECT FOR BATCH COOKING SESSIONS, THESE MEATBALLS FREEZE
WELL. REHEAT THEM WHENEVER YOU DON'T FEEL LIKE COOKING,
AND SERVE OVER HOT VEGETABLE NOODLES WITH NIGHTSHADE-
FREE ITALIAN SAUCE. SPAGHETTI AND MEATBALLS NEVER LOOKED
THIS GOOD! THESE LITTLE GUYS ARE ALSO DELICIOUS SERVED
COLD WITH A SALAD OR SLICED INTO SANDWICHES.

## directions

1. Place the oven rack in the middle position and preheat the oven to 350°F
   (175°C). Grease the bottom of a roasting pan with olive oil and set aside.

2. Combine the beef, pork, coconut aminos, parsley flakes, onion flakes, sea salt,
   and garlic powder in a large bowl. Mix thoroughly using your hands.

3. Scoop out ¼ cup (60 g)-size portions of meat, form into 16 meatballs,
   and arrange on the roasting pan. Bake for 30 to 40 minutes, until the meat
   is brown and cooked through.

4. Serve immediately over vegetable noodles, covered generously in warm
   Nightshade-Free Italian Sauce.

## note

THIS RECIPE IS QUITE VERSATILE, AND THERE IS
ROOM FOR EXPERIMENTATION WITH OTHER
GROUND MEATS (THINK BISON, ELK, OR VEAL).

### ingredients

Extra virgin olive oil for
greasing the pan

1 pound (450 g) ground beef

1 pound (450 g) ground pork

1 tablespoon (15 ml)
coconut aminos

1 tablespoon (1 g)
dried parsley flakes

2 teaspoons (3 g) dried
onion flakes

1½ teaspoons (9 g)
fine sea salt

1 teaspoon garlic powder

Baked Spaghetti Squash
(page 101) or Basil Zucchini
Noodles (page 116)

Nightshade-Free Italian
Sauce (page 38) to taste,
warmed

### prep time
10 minutes

### cook time
40 minutes

### yield
16 meatballs

# TACOS FOR THE MEAT LOVER

TACO DINNERS ARE ALWAYS SO MUCH FUN. THEY ARE THE PERFECT OCCASION TO BRING EVERYONE TOGETHER BECAUSE, HONESTLY, NO ONE CAN SAY NO TO TACOS. THIS FABULOUS AIP VERSION OF EVERYONE'S FAVORITE MEAL ALLOWS FOR SOME "WIGGLE ROOM" SO THAT EVERYONE CAN BUILD THE TACO OF THEIR DREAMS. SERVING QUANTITIES PROVIDED ARE FOR 4 PEOPLE, BUT FEEL FREE TO DOUBLE THE RECIPE FOR A LARGER MEAL.

## *ingredients*

8 No-Fail Turmeric Tortillas (page 32)

**SUGGESTED TACO TOPPINGS:**

2½ cups (120 g) chopped romaine lettuce

2½ cups (220 g) chopped red cabbage

2 avocados, peeled, pitted, and diced

½ cup (8 g) chopped fresh cilantro

½ cup (50 g) chopped scallion

Lemon and/or lime wedges

Creamy Cilantro Dressing (page 44)

3 cups (480 g) Versatile Pulled Pork Carnitas (page 126)

## *directions*

1. If the No-Fail Turmeric Tortillas are cool, reheat before serving. Arrange the toppings in small dishes on the table.

2. Serve the Versatile Pulled Pork Carnitas in warm No-Fail Turmeric Tortillas and top with the suggested taco toppings and Creamy Cilantro Dressing.

## *prep time*
20 minutes

## *yield*
4 servings
(2 tortillas per person)

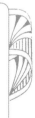

## *note*
TACOS ARE ONE OF THOSE MEALS THAT IS MEANT TO BE PERSONALIZED. FEEL FREE TO EXPERIMENT WITH TOPPINGS AND FLAVORS TO YOUR HEART'S CONTENT.

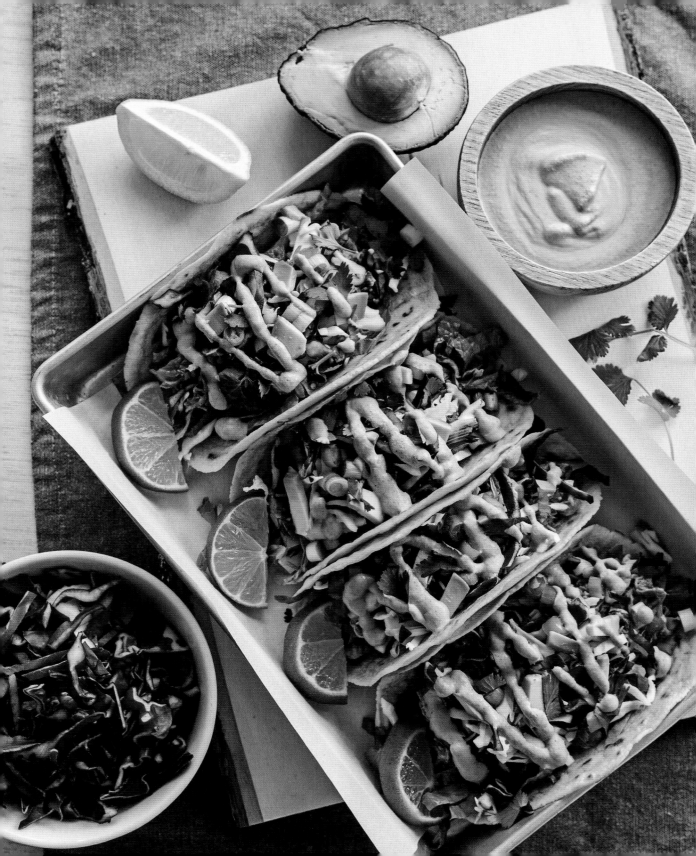

# VERSATILE PULLED PORK CARNITAS

## ingredients

3½ pounds (1.5 kg)
pork shoulder roast

1 (14-ounce, or 400 ml)
can full-fat coconut milk

1 red onion
(about 12 ounces, or 340 g),
finely chopped

5 slices bacon
(about 8 ounces, or 225 g),
thinly sliced

2 tablespoons (30 ml)
balsamic vinegar

1 tablespoon (15 ml)
coconut aminos

1 teaspoon fine sea salt

## prep time
5 minutes

## cook time
10 hours

## yield
8 to 10 (6-ounce, or 170 g)
servings

I CAN'T STOP MYSELF FROM STEALING FORKFULS OF THIS RECIPE RIGHT OUT OF THE SLOW COOKER! IT IS THE PERFECT DISH FOR BATCH COOKING SESSIONS, AS IT MAKES GREAT LEFTOVERS. SERVE OVER CAULIFLOWER RICE FOR A QUICK WEEKNIGHT MEAL, OR MAKE IT TACO NIGHT WITH NO-FAIL TURMERIC TORTILLAS AND A FUN ASSORTMENT OF SIDES.

## directions

1. Place the pork in the slow cooker and add the coconut milk, red onion, bacon, balsamic vinegar, coconut aminos, and sea salt.

2. Cook on low for 8 to 10 hours, until the pork is tender and can be easily shredded.

3. Remove the pork from the slow cooker and shred with two forks. Transfer to a serving dish.

4. Skim excess fat from the reserved cooking liquid with a large spoon. Spoon the remaining liquid over the shredded pork to taste.

## notes

ONCE THE MEAT IS COOL, STORE IN AN AIRTIGHT CONTAINER IN THE REFRIGERATOR FOR UP TO 7 DAYS. REHEAT BEFORE SERVING FOLLOWING YOUR OWN PREFERRED WARMING METHOD.

FREEZES WELL.

*The Autoimmune Protocol Made Simple Cookbook*

# BEEF-BISON BURGERS

BURGERS ARE A GREAT WAY TO GET OUT OF YOUR COMFORT ZONE AND EXPERIMENT WITH DIFFERENT VARIETIES OF MEAT. THERE IS MORE TO LIFE THAN BEEF, PORK, AND CHICKEN. BISON, LAMB, ELK, OSTRICH, AND EVEN YAK ARE ALL EXCELLENT PROTEIN SOURCES THAT MAKE FABULOUS BURGERS. THE SEASONING MIX IN THIS RECIPE CAN SERVE AS AN ALL-PURPOSE SEASONING FOR ALL YOUR MEATS, INCLUDING POULTRY.

## directions

1. Place the oven rack in the top third of the oven and preheat it to 350°F (175°C). Grease a rimmed baking sheet with olive oil and set aside.

2. Combine the beef, bison, shallot, sea salt, basil, cilantro, sage, onion powder, and garlic powder in a bowl. Mix well using your hands until thoroughly combined.

3. Divide the meat mixture into 8 portions and form into patties. Place on the baking sheet and bake for 15 to 20 minutes, until cooked through to 160°F (71°C).

## note

THIS RECIPE IS GREAT FOR BATCH COOKING, AND THESE BURGERS FREEZE WELL. SERVE WITH A SIDE OF SPICY GUACAMOLE (PAGE 39), STRAWBERRY-BEET SALSA (PAGE 37), AND SOME GARLIC REFRIGERATOR PICKLES (PAGE 71). THESE BURGERS ALSO PAIR WELL WITH CRISPY YUCA FRIES (PAGE 102).

### ingredients

Extra virgin olive oil for greasing the baking sheet

1 pound (450 g) ground beef

1 pound (450 g) ground bison

1 shallot (about 3 ounces, or 85 g), minced

¾ teaspoon fine sea salt

½ teaspoon dried basil

½ teaspoon dried cilantro

½ teaspoon dried sage

¼ teaspoon onion powder

¼ teaspoon garlic powder

### prep time
15 minutes

### cook time
20 minutes

### yield
8 servings

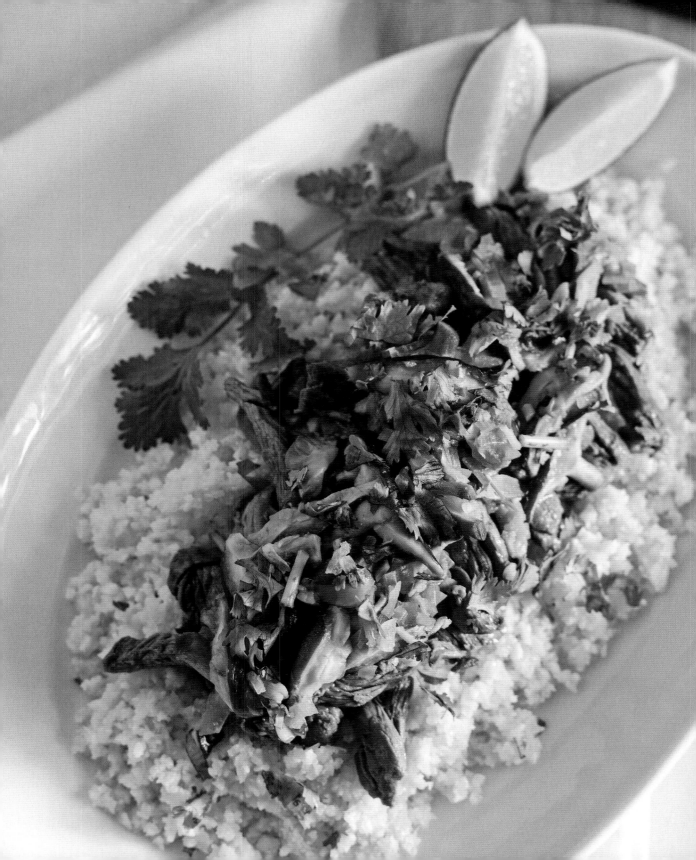

# THAI BEEF

ADAPTING THE RICH FLAVORS OF THAI FOOD INTO AIP-FRIENDLY DISHES IS A REAL DELIGHT. THIS THAI BEEF HAS EVERYTHING YOU HAVE COME TO EXPECT FROM A MEMORABLE DISH—RICH BROTH, SAVORY MEAT, FRESH VEGGIES, SPICY GINGER, AND THAT UNMISTAKABLE UMAMI THAT COMES FROM MIXING IT ALL TOGETHER. ENJOY THIS SPECIAL DISH WITH VEGGIE "NOODLES" OR SPEEDY CAULIFLOWER RICE.

## directions

1. Heat the oil in a large skillet over medium-high heat. Add the beef strips, apple cider vinegar, coconut aminos, and sea salt. Sear for 2 minutes, until the strips are cooked on all sides. They will still be slightly pink inside. Reserve the cooking juices in the pan and transfer the meat to a plate with a slotted spoon. Keep warm.

2. Reduce the heat to medium. Add the shallot and Bone Broth to the skillet and cook, uncovered, stirring regularly, for 5 minutes.

3. Add the mushrooms, ginger, lime zest, cilantro, and Thai basil. Mix well. Continue to cook, covered, for another 5 minutes. Add a little extra broth if the pan gets too dry.

4. Return the meat to the skillet, mix well, and serve immediately with a garnish of cilantro and a side of Speedy Cauliflower Rice (page 106) or the veggie "noodles" of your choice.

## notes

IF YOU DON'T HAVE BEEF SKIRT STEAK ON HAND, SWAP FOR SIRLOIN TIP CUT.

THIS THAI BEEF WILL KEEP FOR UP TO 5 DAYS IN THE REFRIGERATOR.

## ingredients

2 tablespoons (30 ml) extra virgin olive oil or coconut oil

1 pound (450 g) beef skirt steak (or similar cut), cut into ¼-inch (6 mm) strips

2 tablespoons (30 ml) apple cider vinegar

1 tablespoon (15 ml) coconut aminos

½ teaspoon fine sea salt

1 large shallot, minced (about ¾ cup, or 120 g)

⅓ cup (80 ml) Bone Broth (page 34)

6 ounces (170 g) shiitake mushrooms, thinly sliced

1 (1-inch, or 2.5 cm) knob fresh ginger, peeled and grated

Zest of 2 limes

1 cup (16 g) finely chopped fresh cilantro, plus extra for garnish

8 leaves Thai basil, thinly sliced

### prep time
20 minutes

### cook time
12 minutes

### yield
4 servings

# RUSTIC MEATLOAF

WHILE SOME MAY SCOFF, I TEND TO THINK THAT MEATLOAF IS INDISPENSABLE IN TERMS OF FUNDAMENTAL COOKING KNOWLEDGE. IT'S BASIC, SURE, BUT YOU CAN MIX UP THE MEAT, SWAP OUT THE VEGGIES, AND VOILÀ: DINNER! LUNCH! LAST-MINUTE SNACK! IT'S NEVER THE SAME TWICE, AND THERE IS ALWAYS ENOUGH FOR LEFTOVERS. MEATLOAF IS ALSO PERFECT FOR BATCH COOKING, AS IT WILL KEEP FOR SEVERAL DAYS IN THE REFRIGERATOR.

## ingredients

Extra virgin olive oil for greasing the pan

1 pound (450 g) ground beef

1 pound (450 g) ground pork

4 slices (about 5½ ounces, or 150 g) bacon, cut into ¼-inch (6 mm) strips

3 ounces (85 g) mushrooms, chopped

⅓ cup (50 g) finely chopped shallot

1 tablespoon (2 g) dried marjoram

1 teaspoon fine sea salt

**prep time**
10 minutes

**cook time**
75 minutes

**yield**
8 servings

## directions

1. Place the oven rack in the middle position and preheat the oven to 350°F (175°C). Grease an 8½ x 4½-inch (22 x 11 cm) loaf pan with olive oil.

2. Combine the beef, pork, bacon, mushrooms, shallot, marjoram, and sea salt in a bowl and mix well using your hands. Press the meat mixture evenly into the loaf pan.

3. Bake for about 75 minutes, until the meatloaf starts to pull away from the sides of the pan and is cooked through to 160°F (71°C).

4. Serve hot or cold.

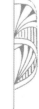

**note**

MEATLOAF FREEZES WELL. DOUBLE THE RECIPE AND FREEZE ONE MEATLOAF FOR LATER.

*The Autoimmune Protocol Made Simple Cookbook*

# BEEF LIVER SKILLET

AIP CONSIDERS ORGAN MEAT, WHICH IS PACKED WITH NUTRIENTS, TO BE A HEALING FOOD. BUT IT CAN BE A LITTLE INTIMIDATING IF YOU'VE NEVER EATEN OR PREPARED IT BEFORE. THIS EASY RECIPE COMBINES A MULTITUDE OF FLAVORS TO HELP YOU EASE INTO THE ORGAN MEAT WORLD. THIS MEAL IS NOURISHING, SATISFYING, AND AN EXCELLENT PAIRING WITH A GREEN SALAD.

## directions

1. Heat the olive oil in a large skillet over medium heat. Add the sweet potato, apple, onion, rosemary, sage, and ¾ teaspoon of the sea salt. Mix well. Cover and sauté, stirring a few times, for about 10 minutes, until tender.

2. Transfer the sweet potato mixture to a plate. Add the beef liver to the skillet (add a few drops of olive oil if needed) and season with the remaining ¼ teaspoon sea salt, the balsamic vinegar, and the coconut aminos. Cook, stirring frequently, for 3 to 5 minutes, until the liver is cooked but slightly pink inside.

3. Remove the skillet from the heat. Add the sweet potato mixture and kale to the skillet and mix well.

4. Serve immediately.

## note

THIS DISH DOES NOT REHEAT WELL.

### ingredients

3 tablespoons (45 ml) extra virgin olive oil

1 sweet potato (about 8 ounces, or 225 g), peeled and diced

1 red apple, cored and diced

½ cup (60 g) minced onion

1 tablespoon (2 g) minced fresh rosemary

1 tablespoon (2 g) minced fresh sage

1 teaspoon fine sea salt, divided

8 ounces (225 g) beef liver, cut into ½-inch (1 cm) pieces

1 tablespoon (15 ml) balsamic vinegar

1 tablespoon (15 ml) coconut aminos

2 cups (32 g) finely sliced kale

### prep time
15 minutes

### cook time
20 minutes

### yield
3 to 4 servings

# ONE-POT CHICKEN BAKE

ONE-POT DISHES ARE ONE OF MY FAVORITE WEEKDAY DINNERS. THEY ARE FAST, EASY, AND REQUIRE MINIMAL CLEANUP. SERVE WITH A LEAFY GREEN SALAD AND YOU'VE GOT YOURSELF A WELL-BALANCED MEAL. THIS ONE-POT RECIPE IS HIGHLY ADAPTABLE. MIX IT UP AND USE SALMON INSTEAD OF CHICKEN, FOR EXAMPLE. OR SWAP OUT THE CHICKEN FOR MORE VEGGIES IF YOU ARE FEELING A LITTLE BIT VEGETARIAN.

## *ingredients*

1 pound (450 g) chopped butternut squash

1 pound (450 g) chopped leeks

1 pound (450 g) chopped turnips

2 pounds (900 g) chicken thighs and/or drumsticks

1 (14-ounce, or 400 ml) can full-fat coconut milk

2 tablespoons (30 ml) coconut aminos

2 tablespoons (4 g) dried sage

1 teaspoon fine sea salt

## *directions*

1. Place the oven rack in the middle position and preheat the oven to 400°F (200°C).

2. Arrange the butternut squash, leeks, and turnips in the bottom of a large baking dish. Place the chicken on top.

3. Mix the coconut milk, coconut aminos, sage, and sea salt in a bowl and pour over the chicken and vegetables.

4. Bake for about 60 minutes, until the vegetables are tender and the chicken is cooked through. Check the seasoning and adjust the salt to taste.

*prep time*
15 minutes

*cook time*
60 minutes

*yield*
4 to 6 servings

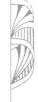

## *note*

THIS MEAL FREEZES WELL. MAKE IT ON A WEEKEND AND SAVE IT FOR A BUSY MIDWEEK TREAT.

*The Autoimmune Protocol Made Simple Cookbook*

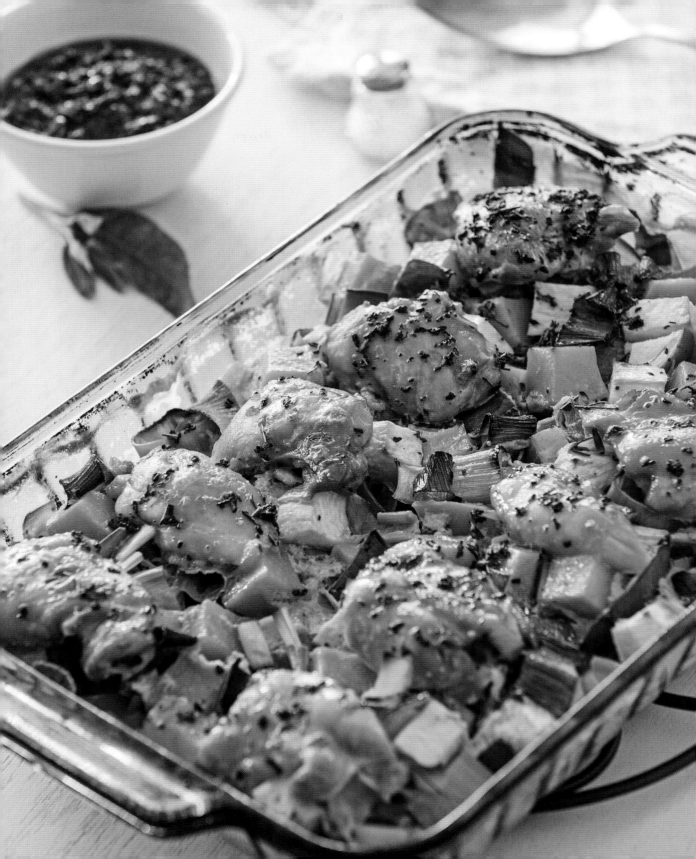

# SLOW-COOKED OXTAIL STEW

STEW IS A CROWD-PLEASER. IT MAY NOT ELICIT THE "OOHS" AND "AHS" OF FANCIER DISHES, BUT NO ONE CAN RESIST CLEANING THEIR PLATE TO A HIGH SHINE WHEN THIS STEW IS ON THE MENU. HEARTY, NUTRIENT-DENSE, AND RICH IN BONE-HEALING GELATIN, THIS SUCCULENT STEW WILL KEEP YOU SATISFIED FOR HOURS. SERVE WITH ROSEMARY AND THYME FOCACCIA (PAGE 31) FOR EXTRA PLATE-CLEANING ASSISTANCE!

## *ingredients*

4 pounds (1.8 kg) oxtail

3 cups (700 ml) Bone Broth (page 34)

2 tablespoons (30 ml) coconut aminos

3 cloves garlic, sliced

2 bay leaves

12 ounces (340 g) chopped carrots

12 ounces (340 g) chopped leeks

8 ounces (225 g) chopped onion

8 ounces (225 g) chopped parsnips

1 handful fresh thyme

1 teaspoon fine sea salt, or more to taste

Minced fresh parsley, for garnish

## *directions*

1. Trim the excess fat from the oxtail if there is too much (a little bit of fat is good, though).

2. Place the oxtail, Bone Broth, coconut aminos, garlic, and bay leaves in the slow cooker. Cover and cook on low for 4 hours.

3. Add the carrots, leeks, onion, parsnips, thyme, and sea salt, and continue to cook on low for 6 hours.

4. Transfer to a serving dish. Discard the bay leaves and thyme. Garnish with minced fresh parsley.

## *prep time*
20 minutes

## *cook time*
10 hours

## *yield*
6 servings

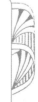

## *notes*

YOU MAY WANT TO REMOVE THE MEAT FROM THE BONES AND SHRED BEFORE SERVING.

FREEZES WELL.

# SLOW-COOKED PLUM CHICKEN STEW

YOU WILL GET A LOT OF BANG FOR YOUR BUCK WITH THIS SLOW-COOKED RECIPE. FIRST, IT IS EASY TO PREPARE AND REQUIRES MINIMAL CLEANUP AFTER. SECOND, ITS SWEET AND SAVORY FLAVOR PROFILE WILL SATISFY EVEN THE PICKIEST EATERS. RICH AND DECIDEDLY DELICIOUS, THIS IS ONE OF THOSE COMFORT FOOD RECIPES THAT YOU CAN THROW TOGETHER IN MINUTES. IT IS ALSO EXCELLENT FOR LEFTOVERS.

## directions

1. Place all the ingredients except the apples in the slow cooker and mix well.

2. Cover and cook on low for 4 hours. Add the apples and continue to cook on low for 2 more hours, until the vegetables are tender and the chicken is cooked through.

3. Check the seasoning and adjust the salt to taste.

### ingredients

1½ pounds (680 g) boneless skinless chicken breasts, cut into 1-inch (2.5 cm) pieces

12 ounces (340 g) carrots, peeled and chopped

12 ounces (340 g) yellow onion, chopped

12 ounces (340 g) sweet potatoes, peeled and chopped

12 pitted plums

2 sprigs fresh rosemary

1 teaspoon fine sea salt

1 (14-ounce, or 400 ml) can full-fat coconut milk

3 red apples, cored and chopped

### prep time
15 minutes

### cook time
6 hours

### yield
5 to 6 servings

## notes

IF YOU DON'T HAVE PLUMS ON HAND, REPLACE WITH DRIED APRICOTS.

DOUBLE THE INGREDIENTS FOR A BIG BATCH AND FREEZE HALF OF IT FOR LATER. YOU'LL HAVE TWO DINNERS IN THE TIME IT TAKES TO MAKE ONE!

# CHAPTER TEN

# SEAFOOD

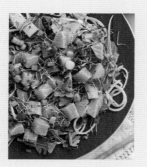

**THE AUTOIMMUNE PROTOCOL** places a significant emphasis on the consumption of quality protein, and although we AIP followers do love a good steak, we cannot deny the simple pleasures of a fresh fish fillet grilled to perfection.

There are many reasons why fish should have a place in your AIP life. It is easy to digest, is packed with beneficial omega-3 fatty acids, and offers a wide range of minerals and vitamins, especially iodine and selenium. Plus, another undeniable advantage of seafood is that it cooks fast. If you find yourself short on time, seafood is a smart choice.

In this chapter, you will find everything from light appetizers to rich main courses. A special effort has been made to favor fish over shellfish, keeping those with food allergies in mind. From family favorites—fish sticks!—to more adventurous dishes such as my wholesome fish gratin, there is something for everyone and every occasion.

Whenever possible and budget permitting, choose wild-caught seafood. Also, check the labels to make sure no food coloring or preservatives have been added (which is often the case with farmed fish). You want your fish to be as fresh as possible, especially when preparing recipes containing raw fish. It is imperative that you choose only the freshest, sushi-grade fish when consuming raw fish. Any dishes utilizing raw fish should be consumed immediately and are not suitable as leftovers. Speak with your local fishmonger before purchasing any fish you plan to consume raw to lower your risk of foodborne illnesses. He or she will be able to direct you to the freshest possible cuts.

Welcome to AIP Seafood.

# TRUFFLE SALT SEA SCALLOPS

RESTAURANT-QUALITY SCALLOPS WITH THAT IRRESISTIBLE CRUST ARE HARD TO IGNORE. THE GOOD NEWS IS, IT'S EASIER THAN YOU THINK TO GET THAT GORGEOUS CRUNCHY CRUST. THE TRICK IS TO DRAW AS MUCH MOISTURE OUT OF THE SEA SCALLOPS AS POSSIBLE BEFORE SEARING THEM. LEAVE THE REST OF IT TO HIGH HEAT. OF COURSE, A LITTLE TRUFFLE SALT NEVER HURT EITHER!

## directions

1. Rinse the scallops, pat dry, and season with truffle salt on each side. Arrange the scallops on a paper towel–lined plate to rest at room temperature for 15 minutes to allow excess moisture to drain.

2. Meanwhile, assemble the salad by mixing together the apple, beet, radishes, scallions, and alfalfa sprouts in a large bowl. Refrigerate until needed.

3. Heat the coconut oil in a large skillet over high heat until the oil starts smoking lightly. Add the scallops (don't let them touch each other) and sear each side for about 1½ minutes, until you obtain a golden crust. You might have to cover the pan with a lid or a splatter guard so the oil doesn't make a mess of your stovetop.

4. Divide the salad evenly among 4 plates, drizzle with the Citrus Vinaigrette, and top each with 3 scallops. Cut the lime in half and squeeze the juice over the scallops right before serving.

## note

THIS RECIPE IS NOT SUITABLE FOR LEFTOVERS OR FOR FREEZING.

### ingredients

12 large sea scallops

Truffle salt, to taste

1 Granny Smith apple (about 8 ounces, or 225 g), julienned

1 golden beet or Chioggia beet (about 8 ounces, or 225 g), julienned

5 radishes, thinly sliced

2 scallions, finely chopped

½ cup (15 g) alfalfa sprouts

2 tablespoons (30 ml) coconut oil

Citrus Vinaigrette (page 45)

1 lime

### prep time
30 minutes

### cook time
3 minutes

### yield
4 servings

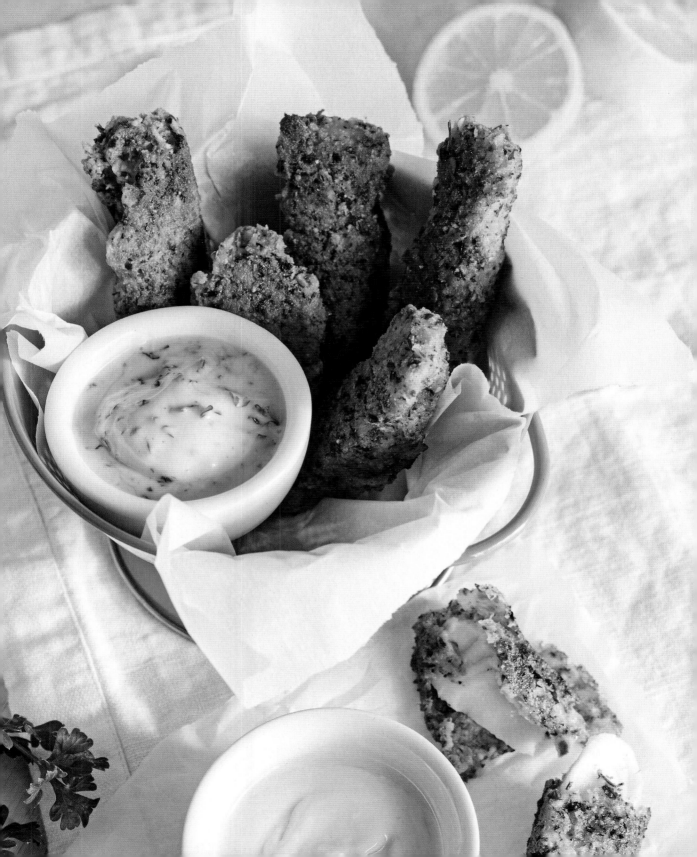

# PAN-FRIED FISH STICKS

CRISPY FRIED FISH ALWAYS SOUNDS TASTY, DON'T YOU THINK? THE GOOD NEWS IS YOU DON'T HAVE TO GIVE IT UP. IF YOU DON'T HAVE A NONSTICK PAN, INCREASE THE QUANTITY OF COCONUT OIL SO THE FISH WON'T STICK TO THE PAN. THIS RECIPE WORKS BETTER IF THE FISH FILLET IS NOT TOO THICK. IF THE FILLET IS THICKER THAN ½ INCH (1 CM), CUT SMALLER STRIPS AND FRY THE SIDES INSTEAD.

## directions

1. Cut the cod fillet into 1-inch (2.5 cm) strips.

2. Mix the cassava flour, tigernut flour, shredded coconut, parsley, cilantro, onion flakes, and sea salt in a bowl.

3. Pour the coconut milk into a shallow dish.

4. Dip each fish strip into the coconut milk, then into the flour mixture, ensuring the strips are entirely coated. Arrange the coated fish on a sheet of parchment paper.

5. Heat 2 tablespoons (30 ml) coconut oil in a nonstick pan over medium heat. The oil should sizzle just a bit. Carefully add some fish to the pan, making sure the strips don't touch. Cover and cook for about 2 minutes, until golden brown. Flip them over and cook, covered, for another 2 minutes. Transfer to a plate with a slotted spoon. If you do this in several batches, make sure you add extra coconut oil each time you start a new batch.

6. Serve immediately with a squeeze of lemon juice and a side of Garlic-Lemon Mayonnaise or Ranch Dressing.

## note

SERVE THESE FISH STICKS IN TACOS.

20 ounces (580 g) skinless cod fillet (or any other white fish), no thicker than ½ inch (1 cm)

⅓ cup (45 g) cassava flour

⅓ cup (40 g) tigernut flour

⅓ cup (90 g) unsweetened shredded coconut

1 tablespoon (1 g) dried parsley

1 tablespoon (1.5 g) dried cilantro

1 tablespoon (6 g) dried onion flakes

1 teaspoon fine sea salt

1 cup (240 ml) full-fat coconut milk

Coconut oil, for frying

Lemon wedges, for garnish

Garlic-Lemon Mayonnaise (page 40) or Ranch Dressing (page 44)

### prep time
10 minutes

### cook time
8 minutes

### yield
12 fish sticks (4 servings)

# SEAFOOD CHOWDER

I DELIBERATELY KEPT THIS CHOWDER RECIPE FREE OF SHELLFISH FOR ALLERGY REASONS, BUT GO AHEAD AND SWAP OUT THE SALMON OR COD FOR ANY OTHER SEAFOOD YOU MAY ENJOY, SUCH AS SHRIMP, SCALLOPS, OR CALAMARI, IF YOU CHOOSE. THE FLAVORS WILL WORK WELL WITH PRETTY MUCH ANY FISH COMBINATION YOU FEEL LIKE TRYING. IF YOU ARE LUCKY TO HAVE THE FRONDS OF THE FENNEL, MINCE THEM AND SERVE IN LIEU OF FRESH THYME.

## *ingredients*

3 tablespoons (45 ml) extra virgin olive oil

3 carrots (about 8 ounces, or 225 g), peeled and diced

3 celery ribs (about 5 ounces, or 140 g), finely chopped

1 small fennel bulb (about 8 ounces, or 225 g), finely chopped

1 small white sweet potato (about 8 ounces, or 225 g), peeled and diced

1½ tablespoons (4 g) minced fresh thyme, plus extra for garnish

1 bay leaf

1 quart (1 L) Bone Broth (page 34)

⅓ pound (150 g) skinless cod fillet (no thicker than 1 inch, or 2.5 cm)

⅓ pound (150 g) skinless salmon fillet (no thicker than 1 inch, or 2.5 cm)

½ cup (120 ml) coconut cream

Fine sea salt, to taste

*prep time*
20 minutes

*cook time*
25 minutes

*yield*
4 (2-cup, or 480 g) servings

## *directions*

1. Heat the olive oil in a stockpot over medium heat. Add the carrots, celery, fennel, sweet potato, thyme, and bay leaf. Sauté, stirring frequently, for about 10 minutes, until crisp-tender. (Don't let the vegetables brown or stick to the bottom of the pot. If needed, reduce the heat or add an extra drizzle of olive oil.)

2. Add the Bone Broth to the pot and bring to a boil over high heat. Reduce the heat to medium. Add the cod and salmon. Cook for 8 to 10 minutes, until the vegetables are tender and the fish is cooked through.

3. Discard the bay leaf and transfer the fish to a plate with a slotted spatula. Break the fish into smaller pieces, discarding any stray fish bones you find. Return the fish to the pot. Stir in the coconut cream and season with sea salt to taste.

4. Garnish with minced fresh thyme right before serving piping hot.

*The Autoimmune Protocol Made Simple Cookbook*

note
_____

COCONUT CREAM CAN
BE SCOOPED OFF THE TOP
OF A CAN OF FULL-FAT
COCONUT MILK THAT HAS
BEEN REFRIGERATED FOR
24 HOURS (THE CREAM
SEPARATES FROM THE WATER
AT COLD TEMPERATURES).

# SEARED TUNA TATAKI

SOMETIMES THE SIMPLEST RECIPES ARE THE BEST. THIS FAST AND EASY DISH HAS LOTS OF TEXTURE AND FLAVOR. THE SOY SAUCE USED IN THE TRADITIONAL TATAKI IS REPLACED HERE WITH AIP-APPROVED COCONUT AMINOS. (IT ONLY HAS TWO INGREDIENTS: FERMENTED COCONUT TREE SAP AND SEA SALT.) BECAUSE YOU WILL BE CONSUMING THE FISH RAW, USE ONLY THE FRESHEST TUNA FOR THIS RECIPE, WILD CAUGHT IF YOU CAN FIND IT.

## *ingredients*

2 tablespoons (30 ml) extra virgin olive oil

12 ounces (340 g) tuna steaks

⅓ cup (80 ml) coconut aminos

1 tablespoon (15 ml) lemon juice

¾ teaspoon grated fresh ginger

½ cup (50 g) sliced scallion

Fine sea salt, to taste

*prep time*
10 minutes

*cook time*
40 seconds

*yield*
4 servings

## *directions*

1. Heat the olive oil in a pan over high heat. Add the tuna and sear for 20 seconds per side.

2. Transfer the fish to a cutting board. Slice thinly and arrange on a platter in a single layer.

3. Combine the coconut aminos, lemon juice, and ginger in a small bowl. Mix well and pour over the fish.

4. Sprinkle the scallions over the fish, add sea salt to taste, and chill in the refrigerator for at least 30 minutes before serving.

## *notes*

SERVE WITH A LIGHT SALAD, SUCH AS JICAMA-MANGO SALAD (PAGE 84), COLESLAW (PAGE 108), OR BASIL ZUCCHINI NOODLES (PAGE 116).

THIS RECIPE IS NOT SUITABLE FOR LEFTOVERS OR FREEZING.

*The Autoimmune Protocol Made Simple Cookbook*

# SMOKED SALMON AND FENNEL SALAD

SALMON IS A FANTASTIC SOURCE OF BENEFICIAL OMEGA-3S, AND SO VERSATILE. IT'S WONDERFUL GRILLED, BAKED, SAUTÉED, RAW—YOU NAME IT. HERE, SMOKED SALMON TAKES CENTER STAGE. DRESSED UP WITH A CITRUSY MARINADE, ITS SMOOTHNESS WORKS WITH THE CRISP FENNEL AND EARTHY BROCCOLI SPROUTS TO CREATE A PERFECT BALANCE OF CONTRASTING FLAVOR AND TEXTURE. ENJOY THIS SALAD AS A SPECIAL LUNCH OR LIGHT DINNER.

## *directions*

1. Carefully separate the slices of salmon and cut into 1-inch (2.5 cm) strips.

2. Place the salmon in a glass bowl and cover with the orange juice and zest, lemon juice and zest, and dill. Toss gently and let the salmon marinate in the refrigerator for no longer than 5 to 10 minutes.

3. Meanwhile, remove the bottom of the fennel bulb with a sharp knife and discard the outer layer. Cut the fennel in half (from top to bottom) and thinly slice.

4. Retrieve the salmon from the refrigerator. Spread the fennel, watercress, scallions, broccoli sprouts, and marinated salmon (with leftover marinade) on a large platter and mix lightly. Garnish with fresh dill.

### *ingredients*

4 ounces (115 g) smoked salmon

Juice and zest of 1 orange

Juice and zest of 1 lemon

1 teaspoon minced fresh dill, plus extra for garnish

1 fennel bulb (about 8 ounces, or 225 g)

2 to 2½ ounces (55 to 70 g) watercress, roughly chopped

2 scallions, chopped

⅓ cup (10 g) broccoli sprouts

### *prep time*
15 minutes

### *yield*
3 to 4 servings

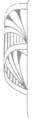

### *note*

SMOKED SALMON AND FENNEL SALAD WILL KEEP FOR UP TO 3 DAYS IN THE REFRIGERATOR.

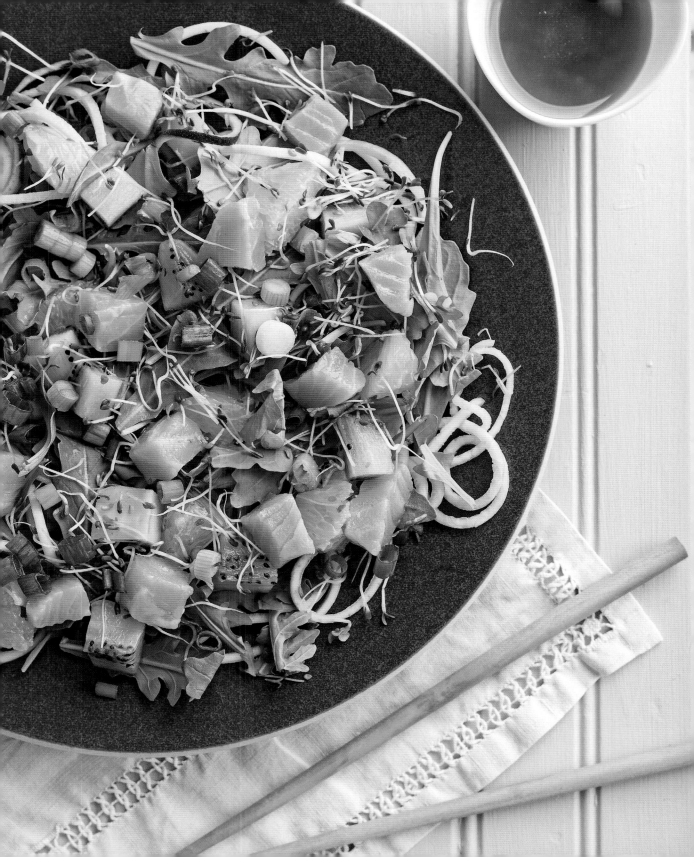

# SALMON POKE BOWL

AH, THE POKE BOWL. NEARLY PERFECT IN ITS SIMPLICITY, THE SALMON POKE BOWL IS SOMETHING I COULD EAT EVERY DAY OF MY LIFE. QUICK, EASY, AND REFRESHING, IT IS A WONDERFUL LIGHT MEAL COMBINING AN ABUNDANCE OF VEGETABLES WITH A HIGHLY NUTRITIOUS SOURCE OF PROTEIN. IF YOU DON'T HAVE (OR DON'T LIKE) SALMON, FEEL FREE TO REPLACE IT WITH TUNA.

## directions

1. Peel the grapefruit, remove the membrane, and cut into cubes. Peel and dice the kiwis. Combine the zucchini noodles and arugula in a large bowl.

2. Divide the ingredients evenly among 4 bowls or plates in the following order: zucchini mixture, grapefruit, kiwi, alfalfa sprouts, salmon, scallions, and chives.

3. Season with sea salt to taste and drizzle with the Shallot Vinaigrette right before serving.

## ingredients

1 grapefruit

2 kiwis

1 pound (450 g) raw zucchini noodles

4 ounces (115 g) baby arugula

1 cup (30 g) alfalfa sprouts

16 ounces (115 g) raw, sashimi-grade salmon, cubed

3 scallions, finely sliced

¼ cup (12 g) sliced chives

Fine sea salt, to taste

Shallot Vinaigrette (page 45)

## prep time
15 minutes

## yield
4 servings

## notes

THIS DISH MUST BE EATEN IMMEDIATELY.

HAVING EXTREMELY FRESH FISH IS VERY IMPORTANT WHEN EATING RAW FISH. CHECK WITH YOUR FISHMONGER FOR THE FRESHEST POSSIBLE SASHIMI CUTS. ASK HIM OR HER WHEN THE SALMON IS COMING IN AND HOW LONG IT HAS BEEN IN THE CASE BEFORE PURCHASING. BUDGET PERMITTING, CHOOSE WILD-CAUGHT SALMON.

# COCONUT MILK SHRIMP CEVICHE

## ingredients

10 ounces (280 ml)
full-fat coconut milk

3 tablespoons (45 ml)
lime juice

1 stalk lemongrass,
cut in half lengthwise

1 teaspoon fine sea salt,
divided

1 cucumber
(about 12 ounces, or 340 g),
peeled, seeded, and diced

1 mango, peeled,
pitted, and diced

½ cup (60 g) finely
chopped red onion

⅓ cup (6 g) minced
fresh cilantro

¼ cup (3 g) minced chives

1 tablespoon (6 g)
grated fresh ginger

2 cloves garlic, minced

20 cooked shrimp

### prep time
20 minutes

### cook time
10 minutes

### yield
4 servings

WHAT MAKES CEVICHE SO DELIGHTFUL? IT'S LIGHT AND CRUNCHY, AND THE COMBINATION OF FRESH LEMONGRASS AND GINGER MAKES IT PARTICULARLY REFRESHING. IT MAKES ME FEEL LIKE I'M ON VACATION. THIS RECIPE TAKES A LITTLE BIT OF CUTTING AND CHOPPING, BUT THE RESULT IS WORTH IT. YOU CAN PREPARE IT IN ADVANCE AND JUST KEEP IT CHILLED UNTIL YOU ARE READY TO SERVE.

## directions

1. Bring the coconut milk, lime juice, lemongrass, and ¾ teaspoon of the sea salt to a boil in a saucepan over high heat. Reduce the heat to medium and simmer, covered, for 10 minutes. Strain the liquid and refrigerate.

2. Combine the cucumber, mango, red onion, cilantro, chives, ginger, garlic, remaining ¼ teaspoon sea salt, and shrimp in a bowl. Pour in the chilled coconut mixture and mix well. Refrigerate until ready to serve.

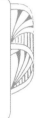

### note
THIS RECIPE IS NOT
SUITABLE FOR LEFTOVERS
OR FOR FREEZING.

*The Autoimmune Protocol Made Simple Cookbook*

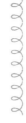

# GARLIC-SEAWEED SHRIMP

SEA VEGETABLES ARE A TERRIFIC SOURCE OF IODINE, VITAMIN B, AND BENEFICIAL DHA OMEGA-3 FATTY ACIDS. THE MOST COMMON OF THESE VEGETABLES ARE DULSE, KOMBU, NORI, AND WAKAME. WHEN COMBINED WITH SWEET SHRIMP AND SHARP GARLIC, THESE BRINY VEGGIES TAKE ON NEW LIFE. STAY AWAY FROM ALGAE SUCH AS CHLORELLA AND SPIRULINA DURING THE ELIMINATION PHASE, THOUGH, AS THEY CAN STIMULATE THE IMMUNE SYSTEM.

## directions

1. Place the shrimp in a resealable plastic bag.

2. Combine the olive oil, seaweed flakes, garlic, and sea salt in a bowl. Stir and pour the marinade over the shrimp. Close the bag and massage the shrimp, making sure each shrimp is well coated with the marinade.

3. Refrigerate, massaging the bag a few times, for 30 minutes.

4. Heat a skillet over medium-high heat and add the marinated shrimp. Toss and cook for about 2 minutes on each side, until the shrimp turn pink. Check the seasoning and adjust the salt to taste. Serve with the Garlic-Lemon Mayonnaise as a dip.

### ingredients

1 pound (450 g) fresh shrimp, peeled and deveined, tails on

⅓ cup (80 ml) extra virgin olive oil

2 teaspoons (2 g) dried and crushed seaweed flakes (see Note)

2 large cloves garlic, minced

¼ teaspoon fine sea salt

Garlic-Lemon Mayonnaise (page 40) to taste

### prep time
10 minutes + 30 minutes marinating

### cook time
4 minutes

### yield
4 servings

## note

DRIED SEAWEED COMES IN DIFFERENT SHAPES AND SIZES. WHICHEVER KIND YOU CHOOSE, CRUSH IT LIGHTLY WITH A MORTAR AND PESTLE SO IT LOOKS LIKE SMALL FLAKES BEFORE MEASURING OUT WHAT YOU NEED FOR THIS RECIPE.

# BAKED COD "EN PAPILLOTE"

DON'T BE INTIMIDATED BY THE FANCINESS OF "EN PAPILLOTE."
IT JUST MEANS "IN PAPER." THE FOOD IS SEALED INSIDE A LITTLE
PACKET OF PARCHMENT PAPER, WHICH STEAMS IT WHILE
PRESERVING THE JUICES AND FLAVOR. YOU CAN PREPARE THE
PACKETS A COUPLE OF HOURS AHEAD OF TIME, REFRIGERATE
THEM, AND POP THEM IN THE OVEN WHEN YOU'RE READY—
CONVENIENCE AND FUN AT THE SAME TIME!

## *ingredients*

1 pound (450 g)
young asparagus spears,
ends trimmed

4 (6-ounce, or 170 g)
cod fish fillets (no thicker
than 1 inch, or 2.5 cm)

Fine sea salt to taste

1 lemon, sliced

2 scallions, finely chopped

½ cup (65 g)
sliced kalamata olives

4 teaspoons capers

4 sprigs fresh thyme

Extra virgin olive oil

Chimichurri Verde (page 43)

## *prep time*
15 minutes

## *cook time*
20 minutes

## *yield*
4 servings

## *directions*

1. Place the oven rack in the middle position and preheat the oven to 400°F (200°C).

2. Cut four 12 x 15-inch (30 x 38 cm) pieces of parchment paper and lay them flat on your workspace with the longer side facing you.

3. Divide the ingredients into 4 even groups. Layer them in the center of each piece of parchment paper in the following order: asparagus, fish fillet, sea salt to taste, lemon slice, scallions, olives, capers, and thyme. Finish with a drizzle of olive oil.

4. Bring the long sides of the parchment paper together and fold several times, sealing tightly. Repeat the same for the left and right side, sealing tightly. There is no right or wrong way to close these packets, as long as they are sealed to prevent the steam from escaping while cooking.

5. Place the packets on a baking sheet. Bake for 15 to 20 minutes, depending on the thickness of the fish.

6. Place each packet on a plate to serve and open carefully. Top each opened packed with a tablespoon (15 ml) of Chimichurri Verde.

note

IF THE ASPARAGUS STALKS
ARE THICK, SLICE THEM
IN HALF LENGTHWISE
TO ENSURE THEY COOK
THROUGH.

# NOURISHING SEAFOOD GRATIN

2 pounds (900 g) parsnips, peeled and chopped

1 (14-ounce, or 400 ml) can + ⅓ cup (80 ml) full-fat coconut milk, divided

1¾ teaspoons fine sea salt, divided

2 tablespoons (30 ml) coconut oil

12 ounces (340 g) carrots, peeled and thinly sliced

8 ounces (225 g) mushrooms, chopped

1 pound (450 g) skinless cod fillets (or any other white fish), cut into 1-inch (2.5 cm) pieces

3 tablespoons (45 ml) coconut aminos

1 tablespoon (15 ml) fish sauce

1½ tablespoons (4 g) minced fresh oregano

prep time
20 minutes

cook time
50 minutes

yield
4 to 6 servings

WHEN WE THINK OF GRATINS, WE USUALLY THINK OF LUSH, CHEESY CASSEROLES BAKED IN CREAM. HERE, I'VE CREATED SOMETHING WITH THE SAME RICHNESS, BUT NONE OF THE INFLAMMATION-CREATING INGREDIENTS THAT WE AVOID ON AIP. THIS GRATIN IS DENSELY PACKED WITH NUTRIENT-RICH VEGETABLES, TASTY FISH, AND SMOOTH, SWEET COCONUT MILK. DIG IN! THIS ONE'S GOING TO MAKE YOU HAPPY.

## directions

1. Place the parsnips in a pot and cover them with water. Bring to a boil over high heat. Reduce the heat to medium and cook for about 15 minutes, until the vegetables are tender. Drain and transfer to a food processor. Add ⅓ cup (80 ml) of the coconut milk and ¾ teaspoon of the sea salt, and mix until smooth and creamy. Set aside.

2. Heat the coconut oil in a large skillet over medium heat. Add the carrots, mushrooms, and ½ teaspoon sea salt and sauté, stirring a few times, for 10 minutes.

3. Place the oven rack in the top third of the oven and preheat it to 350°F (175°C). Spread the sautéed carrots and mushrooms in the bottom of a baking dish. Top with the fish fillets.

4. Combine the remaining can of coconut milk, coconut aminos, fish sauce, oregano, and remaining ½ teaspoon sea salt in a bowl. Mix well and pour over the fish and vegetables.

5. Cover with a layer of mashed parsnips, spreading evenly with a butter knife.

6. Bake for 20 to 25 minutes, until golden. Serve hot.

note

IF YOU DON'T HAVE
COD FILLETS ON
HAND, SWAP FOR
HADDOCK, HALIBUT,
OR SEA BASS.

# FISH TACOS

## ingredients

20 ounces (560 g)
white fish fillets such as
cod or mahi mahi

⅓ cup (80 ml)
extra virgin olive oil

¼ cup (4 g) minced
fresh cilantro,
plus extra for garnish

Juice of 1 lime

¼ teaspoon garlic powder

¼ teaspoon fine sea salt

8 No-Fail Turmeric Tortillas
(page 32)

**SUGGESTED TACO TOPPINGS:**

2½ cups (220 g) chopped
green cabbage

1 cup (110 g)
shredded carrots

1 cup (115 g) sliced radishes

⅓ cup (50 g)
minced red onion

Lemon and/or limes
wedges

Garlic-Lemon Mayonnaise
(page 40)

## prep time
35 minutes + 30 minutes
marinating

## cook time
6 minutes

## yield
4 servings
(2 tortillas per person)

SOME FOODS JUST LEND THEMSELVES TO GOOD TIMES. FISH
TACOS ARE ONE OF THEM. THEY ARE FUN TO MAKE, FUN TO
EAT, AND, THE BEST PART, FUN TO SHARE. SET UP A BUFFET WITH
TOPPINGS, FISH, AND SAUCES, THEN CALL ALL YOUR FRIENDS,
AND THE PARTY WILL MAKE ITSELF!

## directions

1. Place the fish in a resealable plastic bag. Combine the olive oil, cilantro, lime juice, garlic powder, and sea salt in a bowl. Stir and pour the marinade over the fish. Close the bag and massage the fish, making sure it is well coated with the marinade. Refrigerate, massaging the bag a few times, for 30 minutes.

2. Heat a nonstick skillet over medium heat. Take the fish out of the bag, shake off the excess marinade, and cook for 3 to 4 minutes per side, or until the fish flakes easily with a fork. (If using a stainless steel pan, you may have to add some oil to the pan before adding the fish so that it doesn't stick to the pan too much.)

3. Flake the fish with a fork. Now is a good time for a last fish bone check.

4. If the No-Fail Turmeric Tortillas are cool, reheat before serving. Arrange the toppings in small dishes on the table.

5. Serve the seared fish in warm No-Fail Turmeric Tortillas with the toppings.

## note
FOR AN EXTRA SERVING OF VEGETABLES,
SERVE THESE FISH TACOS WITH COLESLAW (PAGE
108) OR JICAMA-MANGO SALAD (PAGE 84).

*The Autoimmune Protocol Made Simple Cookbook*

# QUICK TUNA TARTARE

THIS REFRESHING TUNA TARTARE WORKS WELL AS AN APPETIZER
OR PAIRED WITH A SALAD FOR A LIGHT MEAL. IT IS FANCY ENOUGH
FOR A LUNCHEON, BUT SIMPLE ENOUGH FOR A WEEKNIGHT. ONLY
USE VERY FRESH, SASHIMI-GRADE TUNA FOR THIS RECIPE AND
CONSUME IT IMMEDIATELY. IF YOU DON'T HAVE TUNA ON HAND,
SALMON MAKES AN EXCELLENT ALTERNATIVE.

## directions

1. Cut the tuna into ¼-inch (6 mm) pieces (or as close as possible).

2. Peel and cut the avocado, mango, and zucchini into ¼-inch (6 mm) pieces.
   Thinly slice the scallions.

3. Combine the tuna, avocado, mango, zucchini, scallions, lime juice, and
   olive oil in a bowl. Mix carefully using your hands so as not to smash the
   ingredients. Season with sea salt to taste.

4. Divide the tartare among 4 pretty glass dishes and garnish with chives.

5. Refrigerate for at least 30 minutes before serving. Consume immediately
   after chilling.

## note

THIS DISH IS NOT SUITABLE FOR
LEFTOVERS OR FREEZING.

## ingredients

6 ounces (170 g) very fresh,
sashimi-grade tuna

1 avocado, ripe but still firm

1 mango, ripe but still firm

1 zucchini
(about 6 ounces, or 170 g)

2 scallions

3 tablespoons (45 ml)
lime juice

2 tablespoons (30 ml)
extra virgin olive oil

Fine sea salt, to taste

Minced fresh chives,
for garnish

## prep time
10 minutes

## yield
4 to 6 servings

# CHAPTER ELEVEN

# DRINKS AND DESSERTS

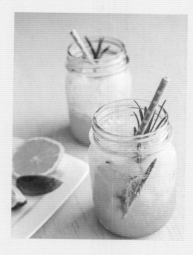

**DO YOU LOVE A GOOD DESSERT?** What a coincidence! Me, too. Despite what it may look like, the Autoimmune Protocol is not about deprivation. I know it can seem austere when you are just starting out, but there is more to AIP than meat and vegetables. Case in point: these fabulous drinks and desserts!

Let me whet your appetite—delectable fruit crumble, fresh trifle, cool popsicles, rich tapioca pudding, and light-as-air mousse. Does this sound like hardship? I didn't think so. Now, just to be clear, this is still AIP. We will still be avoiding refined and processed sugars, dairy, and gluten, among other things. Furthermore, you will need to become familiar with many of the nontraditional, AIP-approved flours out there, such as arrowroot and tapioca, most of which are readily available at grocery stores and online. I know what you're thinking: "How can it be dessert if all the 'dessert-y' parts are gone?" Trust me, you won't miss them. AIP is an investment in your health, but the philosophy at its core is to restore your health *and* your wellness, not make you miserable while everyone else is eating cinnamon rolls.

So, whether you need a little something special for yourself, a snack for your child to share in the classroom, or something fancy for a family celebration, this chapter will provide you with safe options to choose from.

Welcome to AIP Drinks and Desserts.

# FRUIT SALAD WITH COCONUT WHIPPED CREAM

BY NOW, YOU KNOW THAT AIP RESERVES TREATS FOR SPECIAL OCCASIONS. BUT HONESTLY, THOSE SPECIAL OCCASIONS CAN BE PRETTY FEW AND FAR BETWEEN. SOMETIMES YOU JUST NEED DESSERT! THIS REFRESHING AND SATISFYING FRUIT SALAD WILL SATISFY YOUR SWEET TOOTH WITHOUT TAKING YOU OFF THE ROAD TO HEALING. IT'S THE PERFECT LIGHT DESSERT AFTER ANY MEAL, AND YOU CAN VARY THE OFFERING BY SELECTING DIFFERENT SEASONAL FRUITS.

## directions

1. To make the Coconut Whipped Cream: Place the coconut cream and honey in a tall, narrow container. Using a handheld mixer with a whisk attachment, beat the cream for about 1 minute, until smooth and thick. Use immediately or refrigerate for 1 hour for a firmer whipped cream.

2. To assemble the Fruit Salad: Divide the fruit evenly among 4 serving dishes. Drizzle the fruit with orange and lemon juices, and top with a dollop of Coconut Whipped Cream. Don't forget the garnish! Serve chilled.

## note

COCONUT CREAM CAN BE SCOOPED OFF THE TOP OF A CAN OF FULL-FAT COCONUT MILK THAT HAS BEEN REFRIGERATED FOR 24 HOURS (THE CREAM SEPARATES FROM THE WATER AT COLD TEMPERATURES). TO MAKE SURE YOU HAVE ENOUGH CREAM FOR THE RECIPE, I RECOMMEND CHILLING AT LEAST TWO (14-OUNCE, OR 400 ML) CANS OF COCONUT MILK. USE THE LEFTOVER COCONUT WATER FOR A SMOOTHIE.

## ingredients

**FOR THE COCONUT WHIPPED CREAM (MAKES 1 CUP, OR 240 ML):**

1 cup (240 ml) coconut cream (see Note)

½ tablespoon (8 ml) honey

**SPRING AND SUMMER FRUIT MIX:**

12 ounces (340 g) cherries, pitted

8 ounces (225 g) strawberries, stemmed and quartered

1 large peach, peeled, pitted, and chopped

3 apricots, pitted and chopped

Juice of 1 orange

Juice of 1 lemon

½ teaspoon freshly grated ginger

Fresh basil or mint, for garnish

**FALL AND WINTER FRUIT MIX:**

2 pears, peeled, cored, and chopped

2 oranges, peeled and chopped

12 figs, peeled (optional) and quartered

4 kiwis, peeled and chopped

Juice of 1 orange

Juice of 1 lemon

Ground cinnamon or cloves, for garnish

*prep time*
20 minutes

*yield*
4 servings

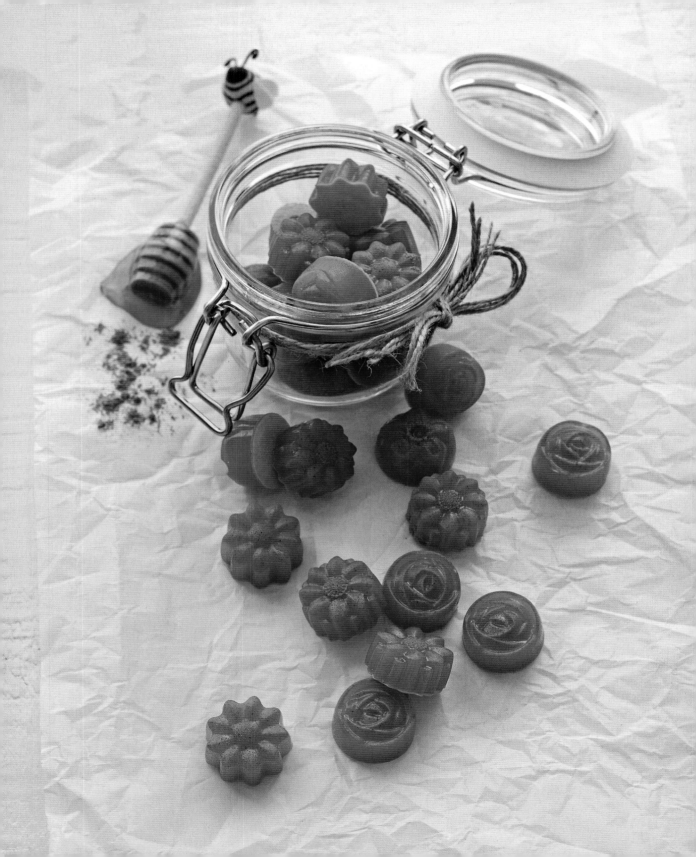

# GUT-HEALING TURMERIC GUMMIES

TURMERIC IS A NATURAL ANTI-INFLAMMATORY AND PAIN RELIEVER. THIS DEEP GOLD-COLORED SPICE, RELATED TO THE GINGER FAMILY, HAS BEEN USED IN AYURVEDIC AND CHINESE MEDICINE FOR CENTURIES TO CLEAR INFECTIONS AND INFLAMMATIONS INSIDE AND OUTSIDE THE BODY. IT IS A POWERFUL ROOT WITH NUMEROUS HEALTH BENEFITS. HERE I HAVE HARNESSED TURMERIC'S POWERS INTO A TASTY LITTLE GUMMY.

## ingredients

1 cup (240 ml) water

2 tablespoons (30 ml) honey

1 teaspoon turmeric powder

2 tablespoons (18 g) unflavored gelatin powder

## prep time
5 minutes

## cook time
8 minutes

## yield
30 gummies

## directions

1. Heat the water, honey, and turmeric powder in a saucepan over medium-high heat, stirring regularly, for about 8 minutes, until hot but not boiling.

2. Remove from the heat and sprinkle the gelatin powder over the warm liquid. Let the gelatin bloom for a couple of minutes before whisking vigorously, ensuring the gelatin powder is completely dissolved and there are no clumps. Alternatively, you can transfer the warm liquid to a blender and mix on high for 20 seconds.

3. Pour the liquid into silicone molds and refrigerate for about 4 hours, until the gelatin is firm. To unmold, push under the mold and the gummies will pop out.

4. Store in an airtight container. The gummies will keep for up to 7 days in the refrigerator.

## note

IF YOU DON'T HAVE SILICONE MOLDS, YOU CAN POUR THE LIQUID INTO A GLASS DISH AND THEN CUT INTO SMALL SQUARES WHEN THE GELATIN IS SET.

# VANILLA-STRAWBERRY ICE CREAM

*ingredients*

**FOR THE STRAWBERRY COULIS (MAKES 2 CUPS, OR 480 ML):**

1 pound (450 g) strawberries, hulled and quartered

2 tablespoons (30 ml) balsamic vinegar

2 tablespoons (30 ml) lemon juice

2 tablespoons (30 ml) honey

**FOR THE VANILLA ICE CREAM:**

2 (14-ounce, or 400 ml) cans full-fat coconut milk

1 vanilla bean

4 tablespoons (60 ml) maple syrup

*prep time*

10 minutes + churning time

*cook time*

20 minutes

*yield*

8 servings

THIS DECADENT ICE CREAM COMBINES THE CLASSIC FLAVORS OF VANILLA AND STRAWBERRY, PLUS A TWIST OF BALSAMIC VINEGAR AND LEMON JUICE. YOUR TASTE BUDS WILL FLIP! THIS RECIPE REQUIRES THE USE OF VANILLA BEAN. VANILLA BEAN IS AIP COMPLIANT, BUT THE SEEDS INSIDE THE BEAN AREN'T PART OF THE ELIMINATION PHASE. EITHER USE THE WHOLE BEAN, OR IF YOU DECIDE TO CUT OPEN THE BEAN, SCRAPE OUT ALL THE SEEDS AND DISCARD BEFORE USING.

## directions

1. To make the Strawberry Coulis: Bring the strawberries, balsamic vinegar, lemon juice, and honey to a boil in a saucepan over high heat. Reduce the heat to medium and simmer, partially covered and stirring a few times, for about 20 minutes, until the fruit is tender. Transfer to a blender and blend until smooth. Refrigerate until needed. The Strawberry Coulis can be made up to 3 days in advance. Keep refrigerated in an airtight container.

2. To make the Vanilla Ice Cream: Bring the coconut milk to a boil in a saucepan over medium-high heat, stirring constantly. Remove from the heat, add the vanilla bean, and infuse for at least 5 minutes. Discard the vanilla bean and stir in the maple syrup. Transfer to a bowl and chill thoroughly in the refrigerator.

3. Once chilled, pour the coconut mixture into the frozen bowl of an ice cream maker and churn, following the manufacturer's instructions. This should take 15 to 20 minutes.

4. Scoop some Vanilla Ice Cream into a freezer-safe container, then add a thin layer of Strawberry Coulis. Continue layering ice cream and coulis until the ice cream is gone. Run a butter knife through the layers a few times to create a marbled effect. Any remaining Strawberry Coulis can be kept in the refrigerator and spooned over the Vanilla Ice Cream when serving.

5. Freeze for at least 2 hours before serving.

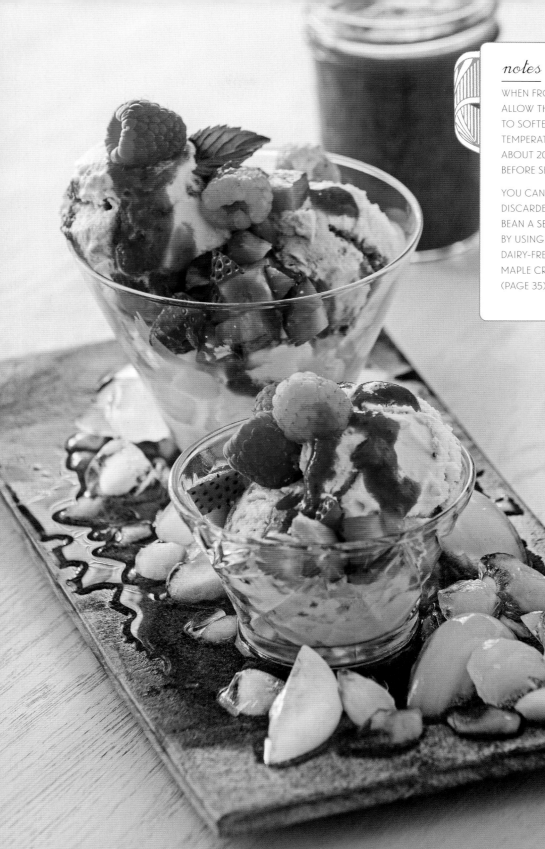

## notes

WHEN FROZEN SOLID, ALLOW THE ICE CREAM TO SOFTEN AT ROOM TEMPERATURE FOR ABOUT 20 MINUTES BEFORE SERVING.

YOU CAN GIVE THE DISCARDED VANILLA BEAN A SECOND LIFE BY USING IT TO MAKE DAIRY-FREE VANILLA-MAPLE CREAMER (PAGE 35).

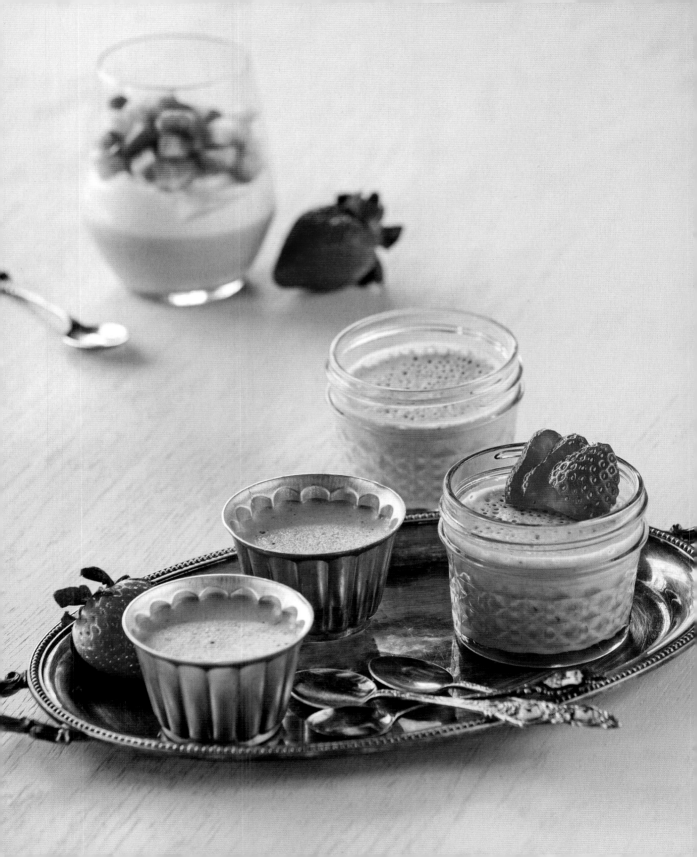

# STRAWBERRY-LIME MOUSSE

THIS SUBLIME LITTLE DESSERT IS EASY TO PREPARE AND REMINDS
ME OF THE STRAWBERRY MILKSHAKES OF MY YOUTH. THIS VERSION
DOESN'T CONTAIN ANY DAIRY, AND THE ADDITION OF LIME JUICE
BOOSTS ITS CLASSIC FLAVOR INTO SOMETHING YOU WILL FIND
YOURSELF DREAMING OF. SUBSTITUTE RASPBERRIES OR BLUEBERRIES
IN PLACE OF THE STRAWBERRIES TO CHANGE IT UP.

## directions

1. Blend the coconut milk and strawberries in a high-speed blender on high for
   about 20 seconds, until smooth.

2. Transfer the mixture to a saucepan. Stir in the honey and lime juice. Heat
   over medium-high heat, stirring regularly, for about 8 minutes, until hot but
   not boiling.

3. Remove from the heat. Sprinkle the gelatin powder over the warm coconut
   mixture and let it bloom for a few minutes. Transfer the liquid back to the
   blender and blend on high for 20 seconds, until the gelatin is dissolved.

4. Pour immediately into 4 small ramekins and refrigerate for at least 3 hours,
   or until the strawberry mousse is firm.

5. Serve chilled as is or with a dollop of Coconut Whipped Cream and fresh,
   diced strawberries.

### ingredients

1 (14-ounce, or 400 ml)
can full-fat coconut milk

1 pound (450 g)
strawberries, hulled and
halved, plus extra for
garnish (optional)

2 tablespoons (30 ml) honey

Juice of ½ lime (about
1 tablespoon, or 15 ml)

1 tablespoon (9 g)
unflavored gelatin powder

Coconut Whipped Cream
(optional, page 155)

### prep time
10 minutes

### cook time
8 minutes

### yield
4 servings

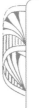

### note

THE MOUSSE WILL KEEP FOR UP TO
5 DAYS, STORED IN AN AIRTIGHT
CONTAINER IN THE REFRIGERATOR.

# TUMMY-SOOTHING POPSICLES

## ingredients

20 ounces (580 ml)
coconut water

⅓ cup (80 ml) lemon juice

1 (1-inch, or 2.5 cm)
knob fresh ginger,
peeled and chopped

10 large fresh mint
leaves, chopped

2 tablespoons (30 ml) honey

## prep time
10 minutes

## yield
10 popsicles

THESE REFRESHING TREATS ARE THE PERFECT REMEDY FOR AN UPSET STOMACH. COMBINING GINGER, WELL KNOWN FOR ITS ABILITY TO SOOTH NAUSEA, WITH LEMON, MINT, AND HONEY MAKES THESE POPSICLES NOT ONLY BENEFICIAL, BUT IRRESISTIBLE AS WELL! AS A BONUS, THE COCONUT WATER PROVIDES AN EXCELLENT SOURCE OF ELECTROLYTES. GIVE THEM A WHIRL THE NEXT TIME YOUR TUMMY NEEDS A LITTLE TLC.

## directions

1. Blend all the ingredients in a high-speed blender on high for 30 to 60 seconds.

2. Pour the liquid into ten popsicle molds and place in the freezer for about 2 hours, until partially frozen.

3. Slide a wooden stick into the center of each popsicle and return them to the freezer for about 3 hours, until completely frozen.

## note

IF YOU DON'T HAVE POPSICLE MOLDS, TRY SMALL PAPER OR PLASTIC CUPS INSTEAD, OR EVEN ICE-CUBE TRAYS. YOU MIGHT HAVE TO CUT THE WOODEN STICKS SHORTER TO ACCOMMODATE.

# TAPIOCA PUDDING WITH PEACH-LAVENDER COMPOTE

THE SWEET SCENT OF RIPE PEACHES ALWAYS MAKES ME THINK OF SUMMERTIME IN THE COUNTRY: FRESH AIR, WIDE-OPEN SPACES, AND THE SENSE THAT ANYTHING IS POSSIBLE. THIS DELICIOUS (AND EASY!) DESSERT WILL TRANSPORT YOU RIGHT OUT OF YOUR KITCHEN. IT IS COMPLETELY AIP COMPLIANT AND SO SATISFYING TO EAT.

## *directions*

1. To make the Peach-Lavender Compote: Combine the peaches, water, honey, and lavender in a pot. Bring to a boil over high heat. Reduce the heat to medium and cook, covered, stirring occasionally, for 15 to 20 minutes, until the fruit is tender and the juice has reduced.

2. Spoon the Peach-Lavender Compote evenly into 4 small dishes. Chill in the refrigerator while you make the pudding.

3. To make the Tapioca Pudding: Combine the coconut milk, maple syrup, and vanilla bean in a pot. Bring to a boil over high heat. Reduce the heat to medium. Stir in the tapioca pearls and simmer, stirring frequently, for about 15 minutes, until the tapioca turns translucent. Discard the vanilla bean.

4. Spoon the Tapioca Pudding evenly over the chilled Peach-Lavender Compote, then return the dishes to the refrigerator for the pudding to set. Serve chilled.

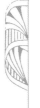

## *note*

YOU CAN GIVE THE DISCARDED VANILLA BEAN A SECOND LIFE BY USING IT TO MAKE DAIRY-FREE VANILLA-MAPLE CREAMER (PAGE 35).

### *ingredients*

**FOR THE PEACH-LAVENDER COMPOTE (MAKES 1½ CUPS, OR 360 ML):**

3 large ripe peaches, peeled, pitted, and cut into ½-inch (1 cm) pieces

2 tablespoons (30 ml) water

½ tablespoon (8 ml) honey

½ teaspoon dried lavender flowers

**FOR THE PUDDING:**

2¼ cups (530 ml) full-fat coconut milk

2 tablespoons (30 ml) maple syrup

1 vanilla bean

3 tablespoons (30 g) tapioca pearls

*prep time*
10 minutes

*cook time*
35 minutes

*yield*
4 servings

# COCONUT-BERRY TRIFLE

I'LL TELL YOU A SECRET: I LOVE TRIFLE! IT'S THE COMBINATION OF TEXTURES THAT I LOVE SO MUCH: COOL WHIPPED CREAM, CRUNCHY COOKIES, SOFT BERRIES. SO DELICIOUS! IF YOU ARE TRAVELING WITH THIS EASY DESSERT, ASSEMBLE THE LAYERS JUST BEFORE SERVING OR THE COOKIES WILL GET MUSHY.

## *ingredients*

**FOR THE COOKIE CRUST:**

½ cup (60 g) tigernut flour

¼ cup (30 g) arrowroot flour

2 tablespoons (14 g) coconut flour

¼ teaspoon baking powder (see Notes)

Pinch of fine sea salt

¼ cup (60 ml) melted palm shortening

2 tablespoons (30 ml) maple syrup

**FOR ASSEMBLY:**

6 ounces (170 g) blueberries

6 ounces (170 g) raspberries

Coconut Whipped Cream (page 155)

*prep time*
10 minutes

*cook time*
18 minutes

*yield*
4 servings

## *directions*

1. Set the oven rack in the middle position and preheat the oven to 350°F (175°C). Line a baking sheet with parchment paper.

2. To make the cookie crust: Combine the tigernut flour, arrowroot flour, coconut flour, baking powder, sea salt, palm shortening, and maple syrup. Mix well with a spatula until you obtain a soft dough.

3. Spread the dough on the baking sheet, pressing down to form a crust about ¼ inch (6 mm) thick. Bake for 15 to 18 minutes, until golden.

4. Carefully transfer the cookie crust to a cooling rack. Allow to cool completely before crumbling into small pieces.

5. To assemble: Line up 4 tall, narrow glasses. Begin with a layer of crumbled cookies, followed by a layer of blueberries and raspberries, and finally a layer of Coconut Whipped Cream. Add a second layer of each ingredient in the same order. Serve chilled.

## *notes*

THIS RECIPE IS QUITE VERSATILE. YOU CAN SWAP BLUEBERRIES AND RASPBERRIES FOR ANY OTHER SEASONAL FRUITS YOU HAVE ON HAND.

MAKE YOUR OWN BAKING POWDER BY MIXING 2 TEASPOONS (6 G) CREAM OF TARTAR WITH 1 TEASPOON BAKING SODA.

*The Autoimmune Protocol Made Simple Cookbook*

# MINI RASPBERRY CHEESECAKES

LIVING WITH AN AUTOIMMUNE CONDITION CAN SOMETIMES FEEL LIKE A FULL-TIME JOB, AND IT IS IMPORTANT TO REMEMBER TO LIVE A LITTLE. SPECIAL OCCASION DESSERTS STILL HAVE A PLACE IN YOUR LIFE, AND THIS RASPBERRY CHEESECAKE IS ONE FOR THE BOOKS. LUSCIOUS AND CREAMY WITH A BRIGHT SPOT OF FRUIT, YOU'LL LOVE THIS CAKE SO MUCH YOU MIGHT EVEN FORGET YOU ARE FOLLOWING AIP.

## directions

1. Place the oven rack in the middle position and preheat the oven to 350°F (175°C). Line a 12-cup muffin pan with paper baking cups.

2. To make the crust: Combine the tigernut flour, coconut flour, baking powder, sea salt, palm shortening, applesauce, and maple syrup in a bowl. Mix well with a spatula until you obtain a soft dough.

3. Divide the dough evenly among the muffin cups, pressing down to form a crust. Bake for 18 to 20 minutes, until golden.

4. To make the filling: Combine the coconut milk, raspberries, and maple syrup in a high-speed blender. Blend thoroughly. Pour the coconut mixture into a saucepan and heat over medium-high heat, stirring frequently, for about 10 minutes, until hot but not boiling. Turn off the heat. Sprinkle the gelatin powder over the hot coconut mixture and let it bloom for a few minutes. Whisk vigorously until the gelatin is dissolved, ensuring there are no clumps.

5. Carefully pour the coconut mixture into the baking cups, covering the crust. Refrigerate for at least 3 hours, or until the filling is firm.

6. Serve chilled as is or with a dollop of Coconut Whipped Cream and fresh raspberries. The cheesecakes will keep for up to 5 days, stored in an airtight container in the refrigerator.

## note

USE THE CRUST RECIPE TO MAKE COOKIES.

## ingredients

**FOR THE CRUST:**

⅔ cup (80 g) tigernut flour

⅓ cup (37 g) coconut flour

½ teaspoon baking powder

¼ teaspoon fine sea salt

⅓ cup (80 ml) melted palm shortening

¼ cup (60 ml) unsweetened applesauce

¼ cup (60 ml) maple syrup

**FOR THE FILLING:**

10 ounces (280 ml) full-fat coconut milk

12 ounces (340 g) raspberries, plus more for serving (optional)

3 tablespoons (45 ml) maple syrup

1 tablespoon (9 g) gelatin powder

Coconut Whipped Cream (optional, page 155), for serving

## prep time
20 minutes

## cook time
30 minutes

## yield
12 mini cheesecakes

# DELECTABLE CHERRY CRUMBLE

## ingredients

**FOR THE FILLING:**

2 pounds (900 g) frozen pitted cherries, thawed (not drained)

3 tablespoons (45 ml) freshly squeezed lemon juice

2 tablespoons (30 ml) honey

**FOR THE CRUMBLE:**

¾ cup (105 g) cassava flour

¾ cup (90 g) tigernut flour

⅓ cup (40 g) coconut flour

½ cup (65 g) granulated date sugar or coconut sugar

½ cup (120 ml) melted palm shortening

¼ cup (60 ml) unsweetened applesauce

Coconut Whipped Cream (page 155) or coconut ice cream, for serving (optional)

*prep time*
10 minutes

*cook time*
20 + 30 minutes

*yield*
8 servings

HERE, THE CHERRIES TAKE CHARGE! PERFECT WARM OR COLD, ON ITS OWN OR WITH COCONUT WHIPPED CREAM, THIS OLD-FASHIONED DELIGHT IS PERFECT FOR A POTLUCK BECAUSE IT WILL FEED A CROWD. IF YOU'RE LUCKY, THERE WILL BE SOME LEFT OVER FOR BREAKFAST THE NEXT DAY, BUT I SURE WOULDN'T HOLD MY BREATH IF I WERE YOU!

## directions

1. Place the oven rack in the middle position and preheat the oven to 350°F (175°C).

2. To make the filling: Combine the cherries, lemon juice, and honey in a saucepan. Bring to a boil over high heat. Reduce the heat to medium and simmer, partially covered and stirring regularly, for about 20 minutes, until the fruit is tender. Keep an eye on it so the fruit doesn't bubble over. Transfer the fruit filling to the bottom of an 8 x 11-inch (20 x 28 cm) glass baking dish.

3. To make the crumble: Combine the cassava flour, tigernut flour, coconut flour, date sugar, palm shortening, and applesauce in a bowl. Mix with a spatula until you obtain a dry and crumbly dough. Crumble the dough over the fruit filling.

4. Bake for 30 minutes, or until the crust turns golden brown.

5. Serve hot as is or with a generous dollop of Coconut Whipped Cream or coconut ice cream. It can also be served cold.

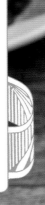

**note**

THIS RECIPE IS SUITABLE FOR FREEZING. I LIKE TO DIVIDE A BIG BATCH OF CHERRY CRUMBLE INTO SMALLER SINGLE-SERVE PORTIONS BEFORE FREEZING. THAW AS NEEDED AND REHEAT SLOWLY IN THE OVEN AT 350°F (175°C).

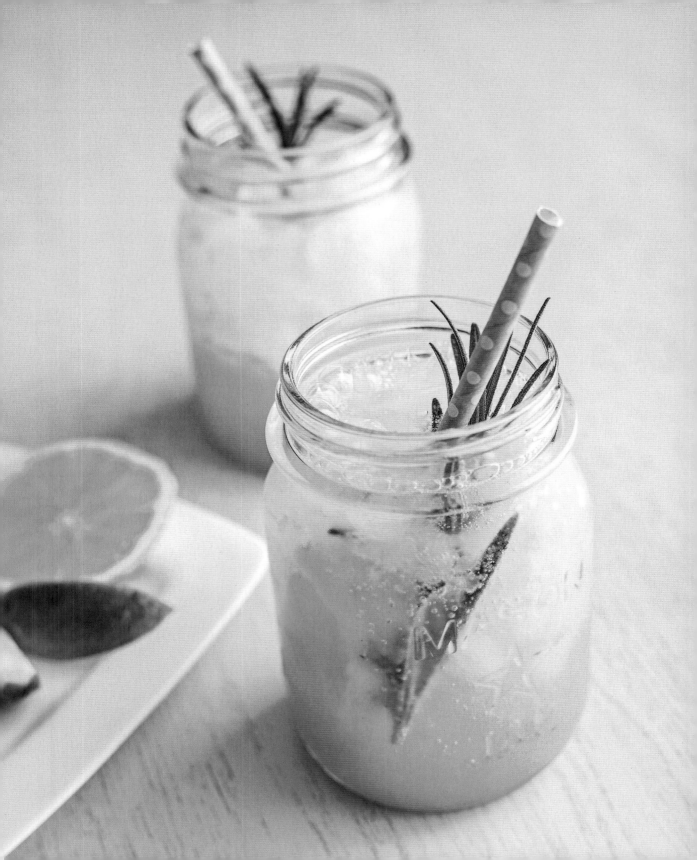

# CITRUS-ROSEMARY SPRITZER

WARM EVENINGS JUST CALL OUT FOR A LIGHT, REFRESHING
SPRITZER. OFTEN, PEOPLE REACH FOR THE WHITE WINE ON THESE
NIGHTS, BUT WITH THE "NO ALCOHOL" RULE IN AIP, WE HAVE TO
GET A LITTLE CREATIVE IN ORDER TO CALM THE CRAVING. HERE
IS A DELICIOUS AND INVIGORATING CITRUS-BASED SPRITZER
PACKING A LOT OF VITAMIN C AND FLAVOR. YOU CAN SIT AND
SIP, ALL THE WHILE KNOWING YOU ARE SO VERY VIRTUOUS AND
HEALTHY. A TOTAL WINE—I MEAN WIN!

## directions

1. To make the Rosemary Syrup: Combine the water, honey, and rosemary in
   a saucepan. Bring to a boil over high heat. Reduce the heat to medium and
   simmer, covered, for 10 minutes. Chill in the refrigerator until needed and
   strain the liquid before using.

2. To assemble the drinks: Combine the grapefruit juice, lime juice, orange
   juice, and Rosemary Syrup in a glass pitcher. Fill 2 tall glasses with a few ice
   cubes and divide the fruit juice between them. Top each glass with ¼ cup
   (60 ml) seltzer water.

3. Garnish with a piece of fresh rosemary and serve immediately.

## note

PREPARE THE ROSEMARY SYRUP AHEAD OF TIME AND LET
IT COOL COMPLETELY BEFORE USING. ROSEMARY SYRUP
WILL KEEP FOR UP TO 5 DAYS IN THE REFRIGERATOR.

## ingredients

**FOR THE ROSEMARY SYRUP
(MAKES 1 CUP, OR 240 ML):**

1 cup (240 ml) water

¼ cup (60 ml) honey

4 (4-inch, or 10 cm)
sprigs rosemary,
plus extra for garnish

**FOR THE DRINKS:**

⅓ cup (80 ml) freshly
squeezed grapefruit juice

¼ cup (60 ml) freshly
squeezed lime juice

¼ cup (60 ml) freshly
squeezed orange juice

¼ cup (60 ml)
rosemary syrup

½ cup (120 ml) seltzer water

### prep time
10 minutes

### cook time
10 minutes

### yield
2 drinks

# HIBISCUS-LAVENDER LEMONADE

## ingredients

**FOR THE LAVENDER SYRUP (MAKES 1 CUP, OR 240 ML):**

1 cup (240 ml) water

¼ cup (60 ml) honey

1 tablespoon (3.5 g) dried lavender flowers, plus extra for garnish

**FOR THE HIBISCUS-LAVENDER LEMONADE:**

1 quart (1 L) water

2 hibiscus tea bags

Juice of 3 lemons

1 cup (240 ml) Lavender Syrup

*prep time*
10 minutes

*cook time*
10 minutes

*yield*
1¼ quarts (1.2 L)

THERE ARE FEW THINGS BETTER THAN SITTING ON THE PORCH IN SUMMER WITH A COOL GLASS OF LEMONADE. HIBISCUS AND LAVENDER MAKE FOR A FANTASTIC FLAVOR COMBINATION IN THIS AIP-APPROVED THIRST-QUENCHER THAT DOESN'T HAVE TO BE CONFINED TO SUMMER. MAKE THE SYRUP AND TEA AHEAD OF TIME SO YOU CAN MIX AND ENJOY THIS LEMONADE ON A WHIM—WINTER, SPRING, SUMMER, OR FALL.

## directions

1. To make the Lavender Syrup: Combine the 1 cup (240 ml) water, honey, and lavender in a saucepan. Bring to a boil over high heat. Reduce the heat to medium and simmer, covered, for 10 minutes. Chill in the refrigerator until needed and strain the liquid before using.

2. To make the Hibiscus-Lavender Lemonade: Bring the 1 quart (1 L) water to a boil in a pot. Steep the hibiscus tea bags in the boiling water for 5 minutes. Discard the tea bags and allow to cool completely. Mix in the lemon juice and Lavender Syrup. Stir well and refrigerate until needed.

3. Garnish with a sprinkle of dried lavender flowers and serve over ice.

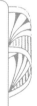

*note*

LAVENDER SYRUP WILL KEEP FOR UP TO 5 DAYS IN THE REFRIGERATOR.

*The Autoimmune Protocol Made Simple Cookbook*

# AIP MULE

EVERYONE LOVES THOSE KICKY COPPER MUGS PEOPLE USE FOR
MOSCOW MULES, BUT AIP SAYS ALCOHOL IS A NO-NO. DOES
THAT MEAN YOU ARE NOW DOOMED TO DRINK OUT OF BORING
GLASSWARE? OF COURSE NOT! THIS DELICIOUS MOCKTAIL GIVES
YOU THE KICK OF A MOSCOW MULE WITHOUT THE ALCOHOL.
YOUR COPPER MUG IS WAITING!

## directions

1. To make the Ginger Syrup: Combine the water, honey, and ginger in a
   saucepan. Bring to a boil over high heat. Reduce the heat to medium and
   simmer, covered, for 10 minutes. Chill in the refrigerator until needed and
   strain the liquid before using.

2. To assemble the drinks: Combine the Ginger Syrup and lemon juice in a
   glass pitcher. Stir well. Fill 2 tall glasses with a few ice cubes and divide the
   ginger–lemon juice mixture between them. Massage the basil leaves with
   your thumb in the palm of your hand and drop into the drinks. Top each
   glass with ¼ cup (60 ml) seltzer water. Serve immediately.

## note

PREPARE THE GINGER SYRUP
AHEAD OF TIME AND LET IT COOL
COMPLETELY BEFORE USING.

## ingredients

**FOR THE GINGER SYRUP
(MAKES 1 CUP, OR 240 ML):**

1 cup (240 ml) water

¼ cup (60 ml) honey

3 tablespoons (18 g)
peeled and grated ginger

**FOR THE DRINKS:**

½ cup (120 ml) Ginger Syrup

⅓ cup (80 ml) lemon juice

4 basil leaves

½ cup (120 ml) seltzer water

*prep time*
10 minutes

*cook time*
10 minutes

*yield*
2 drinks

# ADDITIONAL RESOURCES

**READY TO LEARN MORE ABOUT AUTOIMMUNE HEALTH?** I invite you to visit my blog, *A Squirrel in the Kitchen* (asquirrelinthekitchen.com), for more AIP recipes and lifestyle posts. Be sure to sign up for my newsletter to stay in the loop!

## MORE AUTOIMMUNE PROTOCOL ONLINE RESOURCES

### AUTOIMMUNE WELLNESS

autoimmunewellness.com

Angie Alt, NTC, CHC, and Mickey Trescott, NTP, authors of *The Autoimmune Wellness Handbook* and co-hosts of *The Autoimmune Wellness Podcast*

Mickey and Angie blog about achieving autoimmune wellness through dietary and lifestyle modifications.

### PHOENIX HELIX

phoenixhelix.com

Eileen Laird, author of *A Simple Guide to the Paleo Autoimmune Protocol* and host of the *Phoenix Helix* podcast

Eileen blogs about maximizing autoimmune health through the AIP diet and lifestyle.

### THE PALEO MOM

thepaleomom.com

Sarah Ballantyne, Ph.D., *New York Times* best-selling author of *The Paleo Approach* and *Paleo Principles;* co-host of *The Paleo View* podcast

Scientist turned stay-at-home mom, Sarah Ballantyne shares recipes and explains the science behind the Autoimmune Protocol diet.

## MORE AUTOIMMUNE RESOURCES

*The Autoimmune Wellness Handbook* by Angie Alt, NTC, CHC, and Mickey Trescott, NTP

*The Paleo Approach* by Sarah Ballantyne, Ph.D.

*The Autoimmune Solution* by Amy Myers, M.D.

*The Autoimmune Fix* by Tom O'Bryan, DC, CCN, DACBN

*The Wahls Protocol* by Terry Wahls, M.D.

*Hashimoto's Protocol* by Izabella Wentz, Pharm.D.

## MORE AUTOIMMUNE PROTOCOL COOKBOOKS

*The Alternative Autoimmune Cookbook* by Angie Alt, NTC, CHC

*The Paleo Approach Cookbook* by Sarah Ballantyne, Ph.D.

*The Healing Kitchen* by Alaena Haber, MS, OTR, and Sarah Ballantyne, Ph.D.

*The Autoimmune Paleo Cookbook* by Mickey Trescott, NTP

# ACKNOWLEDGMENTS

**I AM IMMEASURABLY GRATEFUL** to a great number of people in my life. I would like to acknowledge a few of them here.

My family and friends for being my first and best recipe testers, as well as good-natured dishwashers—especially during those exhausting photo shoot days!

Sarah Ballantyne for the groundbreaking work you have accomplished for the entire autoimmune community and for writing the foreword to this book. My life turned around the day I stumbled upon your blog.

Anne Hedgecock, you are my superhero with an eagle eye and magical powers with words!

Lisa Patchem for your talent as a food photographer, your enthusiasm, and your precious friendship.

Andrea Barzvi for your representation and support throughout this process. Your steady presence was invaluable.

Jill Alexander and the team at Fair Winds Press for believing in me and helping me make the Autoimmune Protocol more approachable and sustainable for the many autoimmune warriors out there.

My tribe of autoimmune health bloggers for your daily support, friendship, and collaboration. Wherever you are in the world, I feel close to you!

My readers, who are open-minded, curious, creative, and driven to embark on their own healing journeys. Your constant support and kind words give me the fuel I need to continue creating AIP recipes for your journey and my own.

# ABOUT THE AUTHOR

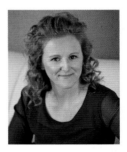

**SOPHIE VAN TIGGELEN** is a passionate foodie, recipe developer, author, and photographer. Diagnosed with Hashimoto's thyroiditis in 2009, she used the Autoimmune Protocol (AIP) to reverse her condition and, today, Sophie lives a full and vibrant life free from the anxiety and flare-ups that often accompany autoimmune diseases.

With her food and lifestyle blog *A Squirrel in the Kitchen*, Sophie shares her AIP experience and empowers others to develop new habits to promote good health and wellness. Through years of experience, she has developed simple strategies to be successful on AIP, including numerous mouth-watering, allergen-free recipes that everyone (even those without autoimmune diseases) can enjoy.

Sophie is on a mission to make the Autoimmune Protocol—and all that it encompasses—more accessible and sustainable for anyone looking for a more nutritious, more delicious, more health-conscious life.

# INDEX